1990

Moral theory and medical practice

Moral theory and medical practice

K. W. M. Fulford

Department of Psychiatry, University of Oxford

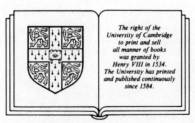

The right of the
University of Cambridge
to print and sell
all manner of books
was granted by
Henry VIII in 1534.
The University has printed
and published continuously
since 1584.

Cambridge University Press
Cambridge
New York   Port Chester
Melbourne   Sydney

Published by the Press Syndicate of the University of Cambridge
The Pitt Building, Trumpington Street, Cambridge CB2 1RP
40 West 20th Street, New York, NY10011, USA
10 Stamford Road, Oakleigh, Melbourne 3166, Australia

First published 1989

Printed in Great Britain at The Bath Press, Avon

British Library cataloguing in publication data
Fulford, K. W. M.
Moral theory and medical practice.
1. Medicine. Ethical aspects
1. Title
174'.2

Library of Congress cataloguing in publication data
Fulford, K.W.M.
Moral theory and medical practice / K.W.M. Fulford.
p.   cm.
Bibliography.
Includes index.
ISBN 0-521-25915-0
1. Medical ethics. 2. Medical care. 1. Title.
[DNLM: 1. Ethics, medical. 2. Philosophy, medical. W 50 F962ml
R724.F861989
174'.2–dc20   89–1026 CIP

ISBN 0 521 259150
ISBN 0 521 38869 4 paperback

US

Contents

Philosophical foreword

Medical ethics is something of a growth industry at the present time; indeed it has been suggested that moral philosophy owes its rebirth, or at least revitalisation, to medicine. Most work in the field is concerned with the examination and solution of practical dilemmas. How long should ailing neonates be kept alive? What are a doctor's duties of confidentiality when one of his patients develops Aids? Should contraceptives be supplied to fifteen-year-old girls without their parents' consent? These are the kinds of questions raised and debated. Dr Fulford's book is quite different. Himself a practising psychiatrist, his concern is far wider than psychiatry. He has a genuinely philosophical interest in the fundamental concepts of his professional expertise.

In the recent past there has been considerable discussion about whether it is proper to talk about mental illness at all. The debate has been carried on in a socio-political context and has been made urgent by the outrage felt in the West by the use of psychiatric hospitals as political prisons in the USSR. Are we not all guilty of treating the deviant as mad; of shutting away against their will people who simply have beliefs different from our own?

Dr Fulford defends the concept of mental illness; and he argues convincingly that there can be a theoretically sound moral justification for committing the mentally ill to hospital against their wishes, in some cases. But in order to reach this conclusion he rightly finds it necessary to analyse in depth the fundamental ideas of medicine, those of illness and disease, first of all in the sphere of the physical, and thereafter of the mental.

In this analysis he makes use of what he regards as the fundamental distinction drawn by moral theory, that between the descriptive and the evaluative (though he recognises that in

vii

practice this distinction is often blurred). He regards both 'illness' and 'disease' as terms which are largely evaluative, though of the two, he argues that 'illness' is more purely evaluative, less descriptive or "scientific"; and that it is the fundamental concept, from which that of disease is derived. Illness is what strikes the patient: the patient is aware that there is "something wrong" with him. Thus evaluation enters right at the start, whether or not any actual disease can be diagnosed. Equally, a patient may have a disease, such as diabetes but, if his disease is controlled, he may not be ill. The notion of 'dysfunction' belongs with disease. To 'illness' on the other hand belongs the more complicated notion of a failure of action. A patient is ill if he cannot do certain things he ordinarily can do. His intentions and plans are disrupted, and he is aware of this whatever he or his doctor may know about the dysfunctioning of his body.

Such a concept of illness makes as much sense of mental as of physical illness. For in mental illness there is also a failure to perform acts that are normally possible, but in this case mental acts. Moreover in the case of so-called psychotic illness, where delusions are present, Dr Fulford argues that the failure is one of intentions or reasons for action. Delusions have often been defined in terms of the holding of false beliefs. However, Dr Fulford demonstrates convincingly that this cannot be a proper definition, partly on the grounds that the beliefs in question need not actually be false, partly because the delusion may not be a matter of true or false belief at all, but rather a matter of attitude or evaluation. And it is evaluations, along with beliefs about matters of fact, that supply us with reasons to act.

It is because the patient suffering from a psychotic illness has a disrupted set of reasons for his actions that it may be necessary, and justifiable, to commit him to hospital against his will. In the nature of the case he cannot both evaluate things as he does, wishing to act as he does, and at the same time see that this evaluation is destructive or dangerous. His doctor's decision to send him to hospital must be recognised as itself evaluative (and of course capable of being disputed), but may be shown to be better founded than the patient's own evaluations.

To give logical priority to the concept of 'illness' rather than 'disease' may seem to make medicine less of a science than some doctors would like to believe. This is not necessarily the case; but it does have the consequence of in part breaking down the barriers between the mental and the physical in illness. Dr Fulford has some important observations about the effect that this might have on the medical profession, and especially on general practitioners. He is also fully aware of the need for further exploration, as far as possible with the help of actual medical examples, of the age-old philosophical problem of the relation of mind to body. The links between theory and practice are here both clear and extremely exciting; and many of the insights are new.

Dr Fulford's book is rigorously argued and the argument is sustained throughout the whole book. It should therefore be read equally carefully by doctors and philosophers, and the arguments examined in detail. There is an enormous amount to be learned from these pages.

Mary Warnock

Clinical preface

The practical context of some of the central philosophical ideas developed in this book is illustrated by the case of Mr A.B. Mr A.B.'s case is described in more detail, along with much further clinical material, in Part IV of the book, Practical applications. It is introduced here to set the scene.

The case of Mr A.B.

Mr A.B., a 48-year-old bank manager, was brought to the casualty department of his local hospital by his wife complaining of burning pains in his face and head. He had a letter from his general practitioner saying that she believed Mr A.B. had become seriously depressed. He had had episodes of depression in the past and during one of these had made a sudden and nearly fatal suicide attempt. The story was that over three to four weeks he had become gloomy and preoccupied and had lost interest in his work. He showed what are called biological symptoms of depression – he had been waking early and had lost weight. He had refused treatment for depression but had agreed to come to casualty to be seen for his head and facial pains. The casualty officer saw Mr A.B. and then called the duty psychiatrist. Mr A.B. was initially very guarded in what he said, but eventually admitted that he believed that he had advanced brain cancer. After a careful neurological examination, the psychiatrist explained to Mr A.B. that there were no signs of this, but Mr A.B. remained adamant. All he wanted was something for the pains. The psychiatrist then saw Mrs A.B. who said that she was very much afraid that Mr A.B. was planning to kill himself. He was behaving as he had done before his previous suicide attempt. As Mr A.B. still insisted that he would not stay in hospital, it seemed to everyone at this stage

x

that there was no option but to admit him under the Mental Health Act as an involuntary patient. He accordingly came into the ward and over a period of eight weeks made a full recovery on anti-depressant therapy.

Mr A.B. and this book

A large majority of those concerned with the care of the mentally ill – doctors, nurses, psychologists, social workers, lawyers, and, not least, patients themselves and their relatives – would consider compulsory or involuntary psychiatric treatment in a case like Mr A.B.'s obligatory. Yet such treatment is highly contentious. Always ethically uncomfortable, sometimes openly abused, it is at the heart of much anti-psychiatric sentiment.

What are the grounds for such treatment? Is it indeed ethically sound even in a case like Mr A.B.'s? If so, why is it ethically dubious in other cases, such as addiction and anorexia? And why is compulsory treatment ethically *un*sound in the case of life-threatening physical illness? Again, if Mr A.B.'s is a central case for compulsory treatment, what makes a case marginal? What diagnostic issues are relevant in uncertain cases? How should discrepancies between professionals be resolved? What, really, should count as abuse of such treatment? How can good practice in this area be safeguarded?

This is not a book of medical ethics, but it is with these and other similarly problematic practical questions in mind, that the mainly theoretical arguments of the book should be read.

Note

All the cases described in this book are based on real patients but with biographical and other individual details altered in order to preserve confidentiality.

Preface

Medicine, it seems, rests on a paradox. It gives every appearance of being a science, yet its key defining concepts, illness, disease and dysfunction, look like evaluative concepts – *ill*ness, *dis*ease, *dys*function. Much of the research into these concepts, notably in the debate about mental illness, has been more or less explicitly from the point of view of the philosophy of science. This no doubt reflects the success of scientific medicine. In this book, however, the medical concepts are considered from the opposite philosophical end, from the point of view of ethical theory. This is a more demanding approach. It is also more rewarding. It produces a clearer and more complete picture of the conceptual structure of medicine, a picture within which both scientific and ethical aspects of the subject are fully reconciled. In addition, it shows a number of new connections between the clinical problems which arise in the everyday practice of medicine and the metaphysical difficulties with which philosophy has traditionally been concerned.

The idea that the medical concepts might be evaluative concepts is not new. Indeed it is widely accepted that in the conceptual structure of medicine there is an evaluative logical element. Many authors, it is true, locate this element at the margins of the subject. At the heart of medicine, it is claimed, there is a body of scientific knowledge expressed by essentially factual disease concepts defined in terms of dysfunction. Wing (1978), and more recently Roth and Kroll (1986), while emphasizing the social and cultural context of medicine, have developed accounts essentially along these lines. Moreover, even those concerned primarily with ethical issues – philosophers such as Flew (1973), Glover (1970) and Boorse (1975) – have often understood medicine in this science-based way. Medical sociologists, on the other hand, have tended to draw

xii

attention to the value-laden nature of lay or non-technical uses of the concept of illness. While Sedgwick (1973), Engelhardt (1975) and others, have argued that, appearances notwithstanding, even the concepts of disease and dysfunction, and these concepts even as they are used in predominantly scientific and technical contexts in medicine, are really evaluative concepts.

The account developed in this book is like Sedgwick's, an ethics-based rather than science-based account. The evaluative logical element in medicine is located not peripherally but centrally. However, the present account differs from previous ethics-based accounts in the form of the argument by which it is established, and, more particularly, in the extent to which its implications are followed through. The ground for this is prepared in an introductory chapter in which the debate about mental illness is considered. Certain features common to the arguments of both sides in this debate are identified. These suggest a wholly new form for the argument which is to come and two outcome criteria by which its results should be judged. The argument proper is then developed in two main stages. In the first stage, the medical concepts are analysed simply as evaluative concepts. In the second, they are analysed as concepts expressing a particular kind of value – that is, medical value as distinct from, say, moral and aesthetic values. The second stage proves a lot more speculative than the first. In the first stage it is possible to draw more or less directly on well-developed philosophical ideas about the logical properties of value terms. This, indeed, judged against the outcome criteria defined in chapter 1, produces a more satisfactory account of the properties of the medical concepts – in particular as they are used in hospital-based physical medicine – than any science-based account. In the second stage of the argument, however, there is no comparable body of philosophical ideas upon which to draw. It is essential to go to this second stage. The requirements of theory aside, many of the clinical difficulties with which the argument is concerned are difficulties not as it were merely of evaluation, but of specifically *medical* evaluation: difficulties about compulsory psychiatric treatment, for example, are often of this kind, as are "mad versus bad" difficulties in forensic psychiatry. Furthermore, the very success of the non-specific ethics-based view developed in the first stage of the argument demands that these difficulties be approached in a similar ethics-based way. But the argument now leads from established ethical theory, and a relatively secure foundation in well-rehearsed philosophical views, into the philosophy of action – not, it is true, in itself a too speculative move: there are obvious conceptual links between ethics and action ("ought implies can", for example, in the well-worn phrase); while in relation to specifically medical value, Toulmin, for instance, has written of "patients and agents" (1980). But here the relationship between illness and action, and the way in which this explains the particular kind of value which is expressed by the medical concepts, has to be worked out *de novo*.

Yet it is in this second and more speculative stage of the argument that the real returns from an ethics-based view start to come in. In the first place, what now emerges is a more complete account of the properties of the medical concepts, in psychological medicine as well as in physical, and in primary health care (e.g., in general practice) as well as in hospital medicine. In the second place, it is with this more complete account that results, not merely explaining the logical properties of the medical concepts, but with implications for actual clinical practice, are finally obtained. Some of these implications are set out in the concluding chapters of the book, drawing on a wide range of examples (mainly) of mental illness, in some instances using actual case histories. Interestingly, it is with these case histories that the implications of an ethics-based account of the medical concepts, not just for medical but also for general philosophical theory, become apparent. The clinical phenomenology especially of delusions, interpreted in the light of this account, is found to have clear implications for ethical theory, and, through this, for epistemology, the mind–body problem, the concept of person, and, not least, the philosophy of science. Apart from ethical theory, the argument in this book reaches no further than the borders of these areas of deep metaphysics. But it reaches the borders of these areas from the philosophically novel direction of the logic of evaluation, and equipped with new data drawn from the phenomenology of illness. There is thus a bonus here. The argument in its first stage involves a contribution from philosophy to medicine. By the end of its second stage there is also a contribution the other way, from medicine back to philosophy.

A few words now by way of explanation. The two-way dependence of the argument of this book – philosophy contributing to medicine and medicine to philosophy – is fundamental. It is from this that anything new in the book is derived. Furthermore, it points to the future development of a true medical philosophy hybrid, in some respects not unlike that which exists, and to such good effect, between medicine and science. However, in the present state of the relationship between medicine and philosophy, the dependence of the argument on both disciplines, fundamental as it is, is a potential communication barrier. Between medicine and science there is a degree of mutual understanding, based on a shared background of knowledge, experience, methods and expectations; and there are of course a good many hybrid medical scientists. But between medicine and philosophy all this is missing and there is thus as yet no common tongue. In this book, then, there will be found rather more explanation of medical ideas than in a purely medical book, and rather more of philosophical than in a purely philosophical book. None of this has to be laboured. The argument being dependent equally on its medical and on its philosophical sources, ideas from either discipline do not have to be explained *before* they are put into use. The explanations are the ideas *in* use. But all the same, rather less is taken for granted than usual.

A second potential communication barrier arises from the philosophical method used in the development of the argument; so called logical or conceptual analysis. The essence of this method – which is described more fully in the introductory chapter – is to explore conceptual difficulties not so much by philosophical reflection as by investigating the way in which the concepts at issue are expressed in ordinary language. This goes back to Wittgenstein. The power of the method comes from the richness and subtlety of ordinary (as distinct from philosophical) usage. However, in order to explore ordinary usage, its component elements have to be separately identified and then labelled. There are two possibilities here. One is to use wholly artificial terms, invented symbols with no etymological connection with ordinary usage: Greek letters are a common device. The alternative is to use real words but defined for purposes of the analysis more narrowly than normal. Neither method is free from communication difficulties. The former because the symbols used carry no "feel" for their meanings. The latter because the "feel" carried by real words may obscure the narrower technical meanings intended. In this book, for good or ill, it is mainly the latter method that is used. As with the medical and philosophical ideas introduced, the terms involved are not defined separately from the argument. They gain meaning in part by explicit definition as they become necessary to the course of the argument, in part from the way in which they are then used in the remainder of the book; 'constituent', 'ordinary', even 'disease' and 'illness' themselves, gain specific meanings in this way, as do a variety of other terms. The way to understand these terms, therefore, and hence the substantive ideas they express, is not in isolation but in the context of the argument of the book taken as a whole.

Note

I follow convention in using single inverted commas where necessary to mark the logical distinction between mention and use: 'x' is thus to be translated according to context as "the term x", "the concept x", etc. Double inverted commas are used in all other cases.

Analytical list of contents

The book is divided into five main sections. Part I is introductory, setting the ground rules for what follows. Part II gives an analysis of the medical terms considered as value items. Part III takes the analysis of part II a step further by considering the medical terms as terms expressing specifically medical value. Part IV is applied: the results of parts II and III are applied to a number of practical problems, especially in psychological medicine and in primary health care. Part V provides an overview of the argument and discusses some of its implications.

PART I – INTRODUCTION

The ground rules for the argument are defined.

1 – The debate about mental illness

The two sides in the debate – for and against the concept of mental illness – share two assumptions and a common form of argument. This is used to show, (1) that the debate is really about the medical concepts generally, not just mental illness; (2) that new assumptions and a different form of argument are needed for this debate; (3) that it should be pursued by the method of logical analysis; and (4) that its results should be judged against two outcome criteria, explanatory power and practical utility.

PART II – ILLNESS AND DISEASE AS VALUE TERMS

The medical concepts are analysed as evaluative concepts giving a view of them which is the reverse of any conventional view, in that, (1) 'illness', rather than 'disease' or 'dysfunction', emerges as the logically primary concept in medicine, and (2) the properties of all three concepts are found to be governed more by the evaluative than the factual logical elements in their meanings.

2 – The conventional view

The basic data – the logical properties of the medical terms in ordinary (technical and lay) usage – is described. The conventional view of the medical concepts is shown to explain only certain of these properties and to lack practical utility. It thus fails against both the outcome criteria pre-set in chapter 1.

3 – Dysfunction

At the heart of the conventional view is the idea that 'dysfunction', although etymologically a value term, is capable of value-free definition. Arguments from the is–ought debate in ethical theory are used to show that 'dysfunction' is indeed a value term. The issues are dramatized in the form of a discussion between two philosophers.

4 – Disease

The conclusion of chapter 3 leaves the way clear for the medical terms generally to be analysed as value terms. This allows the properties of these terms, especially as used in the predominantly scientific context of hospital-based physical medicine (including their largely factual connotations), to be reproduced by summation across the logical properties of a series of hypothetical concepts of 'disease'.

5 – Illness

The analysis of chapter 4 is extended to 'illness', in particular as employed in psychological medicine. The argument takes the form of a progress report, the reverse view of the medical concepts now developed being judged against the two pre-set outcome criteria. It is found to explain more of the properties of these concepts than any conventional view. But in relation to the practical difficulties associated especially with 'mental illness', its main contribution is to raise a question – "How is specifically medical value characterized?"

PART III − ILLNESS AND DISEASE AS MEDICAL
VALUE TERMS

The specifically medical value expressed by the medical concepts is character-
ized by tracing an important logical link between 'illness' and 'action'. This
gives an extended and heuristically more powerful reverse view.

6 − Dysfunction and function

An apparent loophole left in the argument developed in chapter 3 is
used to show that the evaluative logical element in the concept of
'dysfunction' is derived via that of 'function' from the value-laden
concept of 'purpose'.

7 − Illness and action

By an argument which parallels the argument of chapter 6, the
evaluative logical element in the concept of 'illness' is derived via that
of 'action' from the value-laden concept of 'intention'. An evolutionary account of 'illness' is then given in which its properties in ordinary
usage are derived as developments on and from its (conceptual)
origins in the experience of a particular kind of action failure.

8 − Mental illness

The account given in chapter 7 is now generalized from 'physical
illness' to 'mental illness'. The similarities between these two concepts
are traced to their common origins in 'action failure', the differences
between them to differences in the kinds of action failures from
which they are derived.

PART IV − PRACTICAL APPLICATIONS

The practical implications of a reverse view of the medical concepts are
considered for psychological medicine and for primary health care.

9 – Diagnosis

Current classifications of mental disorder remain largely unsatisfactory as a basis for diagnosis in practice. A reverse view of the medical concepts shows that this could be due (in part) to a failure to recognize the logical elements of evaluation and of action failure inherent in these classifications. This suggests a new conceptual framework for future research in this area.

10 – Treatment

Behind many ethical problems in medicine are conceptual difficulties. This is illustrated, using case histories, by compulsory psychiatric treatment. A reverse view (in contradistinction to the conventional view) explicates the intuitive moral grounds for treatment of this kind. Certain previously unrecognized features of the clinical phenomenology of delusions figure importantly in this analysis.

11 – Primary health care

Although its more obvious practical applications are in psychological medicine, the first actual effects of the adoption of a reverse view of the medical concepts are likely to be felt in areas of primary health care such as in general practice.

PART V – CONCLUSIONS

The conclusions to be drawn from the argument are set out.

12 – Overview and implications

An overview of the argument is given. Some of its implications for the future not only of philosophical but also of scientific research in medicine are then reviewed.

Acknowledgements

In writing this book I have received much helpful advice and comment from many friends and colleagues in a number of disciplines. I would like to thank Dr John Bell, Dr Sidney Bloch, Dr Howard Brody, Dr Jonathan Brostoff, Dr R. D. Catterall, Dr Ruth Chadwick, Dr Roger Crisp, Dr Donald Evans, Dr Christopher Fairburn, Ms Philippa Garety, Prof. Michael Gelder, Dr Grant Gillett, Dr Raanon Gillon, Dr Jonathan Glover, Prof. Griffith Edwards, Dr John Hall, Mr Christopher Heginbotham, Prof. Mary Hesse, Dr Roger Higgs, Dr Peter Hodgson, Dr Tony Hope, Prof. Christopher Isham, Prof. Robert Kendell, Prof. Alwyn Lishman, Prof. D. M. MacKinnon, Prof. Basil Mitchell, Dr Catherine Oppenheimer, Lord Quinton, Dr Lawrie Reznek, Mrs Jean Robinson, Sir Martin Roth, Dr Alan Stein, Dr Anthony Storr and Dr Simon Wessely. My particular thanks are due to Mr Anthony Duff of the Department of Philosophy, Stirling University, for his invaluable commentaries on the argument as a whole.

I am also grateful to Mrs Diana Broun, Mrs Carolyn Fordham, Ms Hannah Fulford and Ms Jean van Altena for their hard work on the manuscript, and to Mrs Anne Gray for her help with the bibliography.

The central theme of the book – the application of ethical theory to problems in medical practice – was developed originally for a D.Phil. thesis presented at Oxford. I owe a considerable debt to my supervisor, Baroness Warnock, and to my other graduate teachers, Sir Geoffrey Warnock and Professor R. M. Hare. Much that is right in the book is due to their efforts. The mistakes are my own.

INTRODUCTION

Part 1

I
The debate about
mental illness

Until recently there has been little need for conceptual analysis in medicine. The meanings of the terms 'illness', 'disease', 'symptom', 'health', and so on, by which the language of medicine is characterized, have seemed by and large self-evident; or if not self-evident, at least unproblematic clinically, and hence of no practical importance in everyday medical work. Certainly, if the literature is any guide, any conceptual difficulties which may have been apparent in medicine in the past, must have been of little interest and importance set against the variety of empirical problems with which doctors were occupied. For, with the exception of classical discussions of the meaning of 'illness', and certain later disputes about disease classification, conceptual issues in medicine have traditionally been rather pointedly ignored by doctors and philosophers alike.

But this is not how matters stand now. In recent years, even as scientific medicine has made ever more rapid progress, so clinical problems have arisen which are neither empirical in nature nor susceptible of scientific solutions. The most obvious of these are ethical, medico-legal and political problems, not new to medicine as such, though new in number and in difficulty. But others either raise directly or reflect conceptual issues; and these, as clinical issues, are novel indeed. In the past, for example, the central clinical question, the diagnostic question whether someone is ill, was essentially an empirical question. Whereas now, for different reasons in different cases (several of which are examined in detail in later chapters), the diagnostic question may arise even though the plain facts, as it were, are not in doubt. And in such cases, in so far as it is the meaning of 'illness' itself which is at issue, the clinical difficulties are not empirical but conceptual in nature.

3

It is no coincidence that the progress of scientific medical research should have been paralleled by so large an increase in the importance of conceptual and other non-empirical clinical problems. The latter, on the contrary, has been a direct result of the former. It is well recognized in medical ethics for example, that because there is now a great deal more that doctors *can* do about illness, so there are more, and more urgent, questions about what they *ought* to do. Much the same is true of conceptual problems in medicine. Because there is now a great deal more that doctors can do about *illness*, so there has arisen a tendency to regard an ever wider range of conditions *as* illnesses. Yet at the same time, because of the ethical (and medico-legal and political) questions which have been raised, a tendency of an opposite kind has also arisen; a tendency to *deny* the status of illness to conditions (such as insanity) which were widely (though not universally) regarded as such in the past. And the net result is that the concept of 'illness' has been squeezed between the pressures of these opposing tendencies.

Conceptual difficulties, however, have not appeared uniformly in all branches of medicine. Indeed, although on the whole scientific progress has been most rapid in physical medicine, and although, in physical medicine, ethical, medico-legal and political problems have been evident enough, it has been in psychological medicine that conceptual problems have been most troublesome. Naturally, therefore, the research literature on such problems has been concerned with the concept of 'illness' mainly as it is employed in psychological, rather than physical, medicine – i.e., with the concept of 'mental illness'. This literature, furthermore, has been shaped by the two opposing pressures on the concept of 'illness' mentioned above. It has taken the form of a debate about the validity of the concept of 'mental illness', between those who, essentially, are *for* the concept and those who, essentially, are *against* it. At first the two sides, within medicine at least, were sharply divided. Those for 'mental illness' – mainly establishment figures such as Aubrey Lewis (1955), R. E. Kendell (1975a), and Martin Roth (1976) were unequivocally for it; while those against 'mental illness' – mainly anti-establishment

4

figures such as Thomas Szasz (1960) and R. D. Laing (1967) were equally unequivocally against it. Recently, the two sides have come closer together. Establishment figures – not only doctors, but judges, politicians, health administrators and others – have become more suspicious of uncritical use of the concept of 'mental illness'; while many of its former opponents have come to recognize the validity of at least some of its traditional applications. But the overall form of the debate for and against 'mental illness' has stayed the same.

The differences between the two sides have been widely discussed in the literature (for a review, see Clare, 1979). Not so well recognized, however, though as will be seen in this chapter, conceptually far more significant, are the similarities between them. These similarities, like the debate itself, stem from the non-empirical difficulties – ethical, medico-legal and political – associated with 'mental illness' in clinical practice. Moreover, if they are not well known, this is because their derivation from these difficulties has been so natural that they have passed into the debate, like palmed cards, unremarked. Thus, with these (clinical) difficulties in mind, those on both sides of the debate have assumed that 'mental illness' is (in one or more of four senses to be defined shortly) *the* problem with which they are concerned, their target problem. Correspondingly, those on both sides of the debate have assumed that, in the (same four) senses in which 'mental illness' is a problem, 'physical illness', being on the whole (clinically) *un*problematic, is *not*. Then, taking these two assumptions together, it has been natural for those on both sides of the debate to proceed by comparing putative examples of mental illness with examples of physical illness, concluding either for or against the concept of 'mental illness' according to whether they find mental illnesses to be essentially similar to or essentially different from physical illnesses, respectively.

These similarities – two assumptions and a common form of argument – are most clearly seen by matching the arguments of the two sides step by step. Consider, for example, Kendell's pro-'mental illness' argument in "The concept of disease and its implications for psychiatry" (1975a), and compare this with Szasz's anti-'mental illness' argument in "The myth of mental illness" (1960). 'Mental illness' is identified by both authors as their target problem (assumption 1). Kendell describes his paper as being concerned with "whether mental illnesses are legitimately so called" (p. 305); whereas Szasz, as an antidote to the complacent use of 'mental illness', as he puts it, asks "What is meant when it is asserted that someone is mentally ill?" (p. 113). Both authors then examine a number of examples of physical illness, some of them the same, pointing to whichever conceptual features of these examples they consider essential (assumption 2). Finally, both authors examine a number of examples of mental illness, some of them the same, for the presence or absence of these (supposed) conceptually essential features (common form of argument).

Notwithstanding their contrary conclusions about 'mental illness', therefore, these two authors argue from the same assumptions, through similar examples, and by way of a common form of argument. Yet they come to contrary conclusions. Why? Obviously, it may be said, because the feature of physical illness which is taken by Kendell to be conceptually crucial is quite different from that which is taken by Szasz to be conceptually crucial. Kendell's chosen feature is "biological disadvantage" (1975a, p. 309), or "increased mortality and reduced fertility" (1975a, p. 310). Szasz's chosen feature, on the other hand, is deviation from the "anatomic and genetic" norms of bodily functioning (1960, p. 114). But biological disadvantage is a feature which is shared by at least some of the conditions commonly thought of as mental illnesses, including, for example, schizophrenia; whereas deviation from norms of bodily functioning (such norms having not yet been established) is not. For Kendell, therefore, physical illnesses and mental illnesses are essentially similar, whereas for Szasz they are essentially different. Hence Kendell argues for 'mental illness', Szasz against it.

However, if this explanation of their positions is right, then the second of the two assumptions shared by Kendell and Szasz, unexceptionable though it may appear at first glance, must be wrong. For if, arguing as they do, these two careful authors are able to take quite different features of their examples of physical illness to be conceptually crucial (and a great variety of other features are taken to be conceptually crucial by other authors), then, *de facto*, the concept of 'physical illness', contrary to assumption 2, *is* problematic. Moreover, if – as is the case – their contrary conclusions about 'mental illness' are simple consequences of their different views of 'physical illness', then there is at least *a* clear sense (see below) in which 'physical illness', not 'mental illness', is really their target problem. So the first of their two shared assumptions is wrong as well.

But, someone may now say, the observation from which these two assumptions were so naturally derived, remains. 'Mental illness' *is* a more problematic concept clinically than 'physical illness'. And all that is necessary to square this observation with our new observation (that 'physical illness', although largely problem-free in clinical use, is none the less conceptually problematic), is to distinguish between difficulties in the *use* of a concept and difficulties of *definition*. After all, this distinction is familiar enough elsewhere. Such concepts as 'time', 'redness' and 'baroque', for example, are all normally employed trouble-free. Yet, for different reasons and in different ways, extreme difficulties of definition are presented by each of them. It would obviously be wrong to assume that because conceptual difficulties are not normally raised by asking what time it is, the concept of 'time' is transparent in meaning. Similarly, it is wrong to assume (as has often been assumed in the debate about 'mental illness') that because conceptual difficulties are not normally raised by asking whether someone is physically ill, the concept of 'physical illness' is transparent in meaning. And indeed, our "new" observation shows definitely that it is not. In one sense, therefore, (sense 1 of the 4 to be defined), in the sense that 'physical illness' is unproblematic in use (that is, clinically), assumption 2 would seem to be fully justified (though in this form it is really just an observation not an assumption). In another sense (sense 2 of 4), in the sense that it is an obscure concept, then, certainly, and contrary to assumption 2, 'physical illness' *is* problematic. But even so, and consistently with assumption 1, 'mental illness' is problematic in both these senses.

The distinction which has now been drawn, between difficulties in the use of a concept and difficulties of definition, thus allows us to recast the form of argument conventionally adopted in the debate about 'mental illness' without undermining it. The target problem may now be defined, in a rather more exact version of assumption 1, as the difficulties in use, the clinical difficulties, with which the concept of 'mental illness' is associated. And if, under assumption 2, 'physical illness' is recognized not to be as transparent a concept as clinical appearances might suggest, well, this means only that a more careful analysis of it is now required. But the essential strategy in the conventional form of argument, that of measuring (the clinically problematic) 'mental illness' against (the clinically unproblematic) 'physical illness', still seems right enough. Up to this point, then, merely quantitative, rather than qualitative, departures from the conventional form of argument are indicated.

Once the conventional form of argument has been recast in this way, however, other and more radical consequences appear. In the first place, a definite quality-control test of the argument itself is introduced. Thus, so long as 'physical illness', being unproblematic clinically, is assumed to be a perspicuous concept, it is probable that it will be assumed to be unproblematic clinically *because* it is perspicuous – that is, because everyone knows, or can readily come to know, what is meant by it. And such an assumption is indeed widespread in the debate about 'mental illness'. But once it is recognized that 'physical illness' is in fact an obscure concept, then it must also be recognized that its clinically unproblematic nature rests on some *other* explanation. Of course, to the extent that the use of the concept of 'physical illness' happens to *be* problem-free in everyday clinical work in physical medicine, there is no need, for practical purposes, to explain *why* it is problem-free. But if the concept of 'physical illness' is to be employed as in the conventional form of argument, then some explanation of its clinically unproblematic nature is required. Otherwise, the "careful" analysis of it, which has now been found to be necessary, will be seriously incomplete. Hence our quality-control test. For we now see that the stage of the conventional form of argument at which the concept of 'physical illness' is analysed is incomplete (and the argument, therefore, suspect) unless and until some explanation is found for the fact that, although obscure in meaning, the concept is none the less problem-free in clinical use.

A first such explanation which may spring to mind is that 'physical illness', although an obscure concept, is for all that (in some sense or other) a *sound* concept. Certainly, such an explanation would be attractive to those who would argue along conventional lines. For unless 'physical illness' is taken at least to be a more sound concept than 'mental illness', there is no justification for making 'physical illness' the measure of 'mental illness'. Indeed, in the debate about 'mental illness', this idea, that 'physical illness' is conceptually sound, commonly figures as a variant of assumption 2 – 'physical illness', it is assumed, is unproblematic in the sense (sense 3 of 4) that, obscure in meaning or not, it is (somehow) conceptually sound. And this assumption may seem both to be supported by and to explain the fact that the use of the concept is to so large an extent problem-free.

However, that 'physical illness' is sound conceptually cannot, in advance of analysis, just be assumed. Nor, in advance of analysis, can the fact that it is problem-free in use be adduced as evidence that it is conceptually sound. For this fact could be explained in a number of other, and quite different, ways. It could be, for example, that although the concept of 'physical illness', as normally employed, is actually a *defective* concept, the circumstances in which it is normally employed are such that its defects are not apparent; or that, though they are apparent, they are not recognized; or that, though recognized, they are suppressed or ignored. Ironically, if 'physical illness' were transparent in meaning, it might be possible to choose between different explanations of its clinically unproblematic nature by direct inspection, as it were. But it is not transparent in meaning. In the conventional form of argument as it has now been recast, therefore, the conceptual soundness of 'physical illness', far from being assumed must be demonstrated, and demonstrated against competing explanations of its clinically unproblematic nature. Thus is introduced, as a second consequence of our recasting of the conventional form of argument, a second quality-control test of the argument itself.

Still, it may now be said, counter-attacking once more on behalf of the conventional form of argument, something crucial has been left out of the foregoing account – namely, the particular *kind* of clinical difficulty which is associated with 'mental illness' (and from which 'physical illness' is largely free), the 'diagnostic' difficulty mentioned earlier. For the foundation of the conventional form of argument is not that 'physical illness' is, in some non-specific way, problem-free compared with 'mental illness', but that it is free from problems of this particular kind.

To see that this is so, this counter-attack might continue, we need only compare the "diagnostic" difficulty itself as it arises in respect of the two kinds of illness. If a patient is diagnosed as suffering from a condition such as true or classical migraine (defined by pain of a relapsing character in one half of the head, visual disturbance, photophobia, sickness, and so on), it will be taken for granted in practice that the patient is (physically) ill. At all events, the diagnostic question "Is the patient ill?", although in principle separable from the diagnostic question "What condition is he suffering from?", will normally have no practical clinical significance whatsoever. In the case of migraine, therefore, and of most similar conditions, the former diagnosis, the "illness-diagnosis" as it were, has in effect already been made once the latter, or "condition-diagnosis", has been made.

But now compare this with a condition such as depression. If a patient is diagnosed as suffering from depression, the further diagnostic question, the illness-diagnostic question – whether, thereby, the patient is ill – will remain an open, and often clinically important, question. Compulsory medical treatment, for example, (which is considered in chapter 10) is justified, ethically and legally, only if the patient in question, being depressed, is thereby ill. Moreover, it is with questions of this latter kind, illness-diagnostic questions, or with the general question to which such questions give rise, that the debate about 'mental illness' is centrally concerned – with whether, in Kendell's words again, "mental illnesses are legitimately so called". And it is because questions of this kind are not normally raised by conditions such as migraine that it surely makes good sense to proceed, as in the conventional form of argument, by comparing putative mental illnesses with these conditions. For to say that it can be taken for granted that patients with conditions such as migraine are ill, is just another way of saying that it can be taken for granted that conditions such as migraine really *are* illnesses. It may thus be readily admitted that a more careful analysis of the concept of 'physical illness' is required than has hitherto been carried out. It may even be admitted that the concept of 'physical illness', as normally employed, is not without defects. But if conditions such as migraine really *are* illnesses, then by comparing conditions like depression with them, it should in principle be possible to decide the illness-diagnostic question with which the debate about 'mental illness' is ultimately concerned – namely, whether conditions of this latter kind are also really illnesses. However, it is precisely this comparison which is at the heart of the conventional form of argument. Therefore, this counter-attack concludes, is not the conventional form of argument fully justified?

There is much in this tidied-up version of the conventional form of argument with which it is possible to agree. To start from examples of physical illness is clearly a sound strategy. If nothing else, such examples provide common ground between the two sides in the debate about 'mental illness'. And an analysis of examples of this kind is thus likely to be an important step on the route to conclusions about 'mental illness'. There are, however, other routes from examples of physical illness to conclusions about 'mental illness'. There are, indeed, better routes. For the conventional route involves a slide, a conceptual slide from the concept of 'physical illness' to the more general concept, 'illness'.

In the conventional form of argument, as has been seen, putative examples of mental illness are compared more or less directly with examples of physical illness, to determine, essentially, whether or not the former show whichever feature of the latter the particular author has taken to be conceptually crucial. However, as this form of argument is normally developed, it is not made clear whether the (supposed) conceptually crucial feature is taken to be crucial to the general concept 'illness' or just to the particular concept 'physical illness'. Indeed, in the literature, these two concepts tend not to be distinguished explicitly at all. From the fact that the comparison is in general a more or less direct comparison of examples of mental illness with those of physical illness, it would seem that it is the concept of 'physical illness' which most authors have in mind. But if so, then, strictly speaking, such a comparison can show only that mental illnesses either are (because they are essentially similar to) or are not (because they are essentially different from) *physical* illnesses; whereas the conclusions of the conventional form of argument as conventionally expressed are that mental illnesses either are or are not *illnesses* in their own right. Kendell's pro-'mental illness' conclusion, for example, is that *mental* illnesses are legitimately so called – that is, they are mental, not physical, illnesses; whereas Szasz's anti-'mental-illness' conclusion is simply that mental illnesses are not *illnesses* at all. But conclusions such as these could only be drawn by measuring (putative) mental illnesses against the concept of 'illness'.

It is not difficult to see how this slide comes about. In the first place, since it is only conditions such as migraine which can be taken for granted as real illnesses, and since conditions such as migraine are ordinarily thought of as physical illnesses, the two concepts, 'illness' and 'physical illness', can easily be conflated. Then again, there is an obvious temptation, even if the two concepts are carefully distinguished, to suppose that examples of physical illness are somehow more central or more authentic examples of illness than are examples of mental illness. Certainly, in the debate about 'mental illness', some such assumption is a common enough variant of assumption 2: the sense (sense 4 of 4) in which 'physical illness' is assumed to be unproblematic is then that, obscure in meaning or not, defective in other ways or not, examples of it are, at the very least, authentic examples of illness. But this, combined with the corresponding contrary assumption about 'mental illness', comes close to assuming that everyone who is authentically ill is physically ill; and hence that the terms 'illness' and 'physical illness' are coextensive as regards the conditions to which they may properly be applied. This, in turn, comes close to assuming that these two terms are near, if not actual, synonyms – for if they are indeed coextensive in application, while they could still in principle be distinct in meaning (they could, for example, mark out different features of the conditions to which they were jointly and severally applicable), there would be that much less point in distinguishing between them. In which case they would not often be distinguished. And they would thus, being often used as synonyms, come to be thought of *as* synonyms. Hence a slide from one to the other, as in the conventional form of argument, would seem not only possible, but to a large extent justified.

This could be right, of course. It could be that the terms 'illness' and 'physical illness', are not (or not significantly) different in meaning. It could be that there is no general concept 'illness', distinct from (or significantly distinct from) the particular concept 'physical illness'. However, since a (significantly) distinct general concept is implied by *talk* of two kinds of illness, physical illness and mental illness, it certainly cannot be taken for granted that there is none. Indeed, since the legitimacy of such talk is dependent (*inter alia*, as we will see below) on there being such a concept, and since it is with the legitimacy of such talk that the debate about 'mental illness' is concerned, far from it being assumed in the debate that 'illness' and 'physical illness' are essentially the same, a central objective of the debate itself must be to determine whether in fact this is so.

We have thus arrived at a third and more drastic consequence of recasting the conventional form of argument. For it has now been found that if, from examples of physical illness, conclusions of a conventional kind are to be drawn about 'mental illness', the route from the former to the latter must be qualitatively, and not merely quantitatively, different from that which is conventionally adopted. Instead of putative examples of mental illness being measured against examples of physical illness (with some conflation of the concepts of 'illness' and 'physical illness' in mind), it must first be determined (by analyses of examples of physical illness or in any other way) whether there is a general concept, 'illness', distinct from

13

'physical illness'. If there is not, then the form of argument reverts to convention, with putative examples of mental illness being measured against the concept of 'physical illness'; though now with a clear recognition that the conclusions to be drawn thereby are the *un*conventional conclusions noted a moment ago, that mental illnesses either are or are not *physical* illnesses. If, on the other hand, it turns out that there is a distinct general concept (and at this stage, of course, in advance of analysis, nothing can be said about what such a concept would consist in), then the argument can proceed quite differently – namely, as will be described in more detail later on, by generalization rather than direct comparison. For then, instead of putative mental illnesses being measured against examples of physical illnesses, they could be measured against the general concept 'illness'. And the conclusions which would then be drawn would be the conventional conclusions that mental illnesses either are or are not illnesses in their own right.

An immediate caveat is necessary, however. The mere finding of a distinct general concept in itself provides no guarantee of the validity of the concept of 'mental illness'. To decide this (one way or the other), the authenticity of individual putative examples of mental illness would still have to be established, by carefully measuring them against the general concept 'illness'. Moreover, given the great variety of putative mental illnesses currently extant, it is likely that some of these will fail to measure up satisfactorily. And to the extent of such failures, the scope of the concept of 'mental illness', as currently employed, would be diminished. On the other hand, it could end up enlarged, with conditions not previously recognized as mental illnesses being found to be so. At all events, if a general concept *is* found, it is highly likely that at least some conditions will prove to be authentic mental illnesses, for otherwise it is hard to imagine why there should be a general concept at all. But even this cannot be taken for granted. For the generalization implied by the existence of a distinct general concept could be in some other, perhaps as yet wholly unrecognized direction. Furthermore, even though some of the conditions currently thought of as mental illnesses turn out authentically to be so, the precise sense in which they are illnesses – let alone the sense in which they are mental illnesses – might prove to be very different from the senses of these terms as ordinarily understood. Then again, just as the concept of 'physical illness', as ordinarily employed, may in certain respects be defective, so also may the concept of 'mental illness'. Therefore, even though some mental illnesses may prove to be (in Kendell's phrase) legitimately so called, and even though (contrary to Szasz's conclusion) at least some mental illnesses may prove to be authentic examples of illness, yet the concept of 'mental illness', *post* analysis as it were, may be understood quite differently from the way in which it is currently understood. A valid concept it may thus prove to be, but at the expense, rather than in vindication, of ordinary understanding.

There is thus, if the argument proceeds by generalization, much scope for complications. Any conclusions reached about 'mental illness' are unlikely to be of the crisp, dogmatic kind familiar in so much of the literature. Not, however, that similar complications are in any way disallowed in the conventional form of argument by direct comparison. On the contrary, they are more than likely to be there, once it is recognized that the concept of 'physical illness' is a far from perspicuous concept, requiring assiduous analysis in its own right. Indeed once this is recognized, it becomes clear that 'physical illness' itself is unlikely to be as neat, as clean-cut, as well circumscribed a concept as in the debate about 'mental illness' it has generally been taken to be. And if this is true of 'physical illness', how much more so will it be for any general concept of 'illness' which can be distinguished from it. Not only that, but both concepts, 'physical illness' and 'illness', may well turn out not to be single concepts at all, but families of overlapping or otherwise interrelated concepts, each of which in its own right may be intricate, subtle and obscure.

Imagine, then, the potential difficulties when, drawing on results derived from either form of argument (by generalization or by direct comparison), individual clinical cases are considered. To the illness-diagnostic question, simple enough to frame, there are likely to be no simple answers. In the first place, however clearly and completely the possible senses of 'illness', 'mental illness' and 'physical illness' have all been defined, difficulties in the actual use of these terms could still arise. Fine distinctions, for example, or problematic judgements could be implied by them; or they could be just plain complicated. Then, if indeed each term has a number of distinct senses, an illness-diagnosis in respect of just one given condition could be constituted by any of the possible combinations of these senses. Hence a given patient, suffering from only one condition, could legitimately be found to be both ill (in some senses of the term) and yet not ill (in other senses of the term). Similarly, the patient could be found to be (in different senses of the respective terms) both mentally ill and yet not mentally ill, physically ill and yet not physically ill; even (in virtue only of that one condition, remember) both mentally ill and physically ill, the distinction between these two kinds of illness becoming thereby that much less clearcut.

Nor do the potential difficulties end here. For a quite distinct third kind of difficulty could arise if it turned out that the legitimacy with which a patient may be said to be ill (and/or mentally ill, and/or physically ill) is dependent on considerations other than just the features of the condition from which he or she is suffering. It could be, for example, that, in one or more of its senses, the concept of 'illness' is such that, besides the condition of the patient, the circumstances in which an illness-diagnosis is made – even the purposes for which it is made – are relevant to the diagnosis. If so, then illness-diagnostic opinion would legitimately be more diverse than condition-diagnostic opinion. For different doctors, let alone professionals of other kinds, let alone non-professionals such as patients themselves or their relatives, could legitimately come to different illness-diagnostic opinions, even employing the *same* sense of illness, in respect of the *same* patient, and granted the *same* condition-diagnosis.

It might be hoped, from a clinical point of view, that matters will not turn out as difficult as all that! But from the point of view of analysis, such difficulties hardly present a gloomy prospect; for they are, after all, broadly consonant with clinical experience. In actual clinical practice, mental illness and physical illness are simply not the sharply distinct kinds of illness so

commonly portrayed in the literature. And we should certainly not need to be reminded of the difficulties presented by
illness-diagnosis, nor of the diversity of illness-diagnostic
opinion, since these are among the very non-empirical clinical
problems with which, as was seen at the start of this chapter,
analytical research in medicine is centrally concerned.

Furthermore, if it is considered that these diagnostic difficulties and this diversity of diagnostic opinion are only provisionally legitimate, it is far from obvious that their legitimacy is
provisional (as it would be in the case of condition-diagnoses)
only on a deeper or more extensive knowledge of fact. This is
most obviously so where the issues at stake in diagnosis include
such weighty ethical and medico-legal matters as compulsory
psychiatric treatment, criminal responsibility and civil capacity. But it is true also in more everyday general medical
contexts, such as the issuing of "off-work" certificates or
reporting for insurance purposes. In all such instances, it is a
matter of observation that illness-diagnostic opinion is often
diverse. And it is a matter of observation also that this diversity
is not due, or due solely, to diversity of condition-diagnostic
opinion (since the condition of the patient is often not at issue
at all). Then again, although in such instances expert medical
opinion is always important, it is not always regarded (as in
respect of condition-diagnoses it would be regarded) as decisive. In court proceedings, for example, medical opinion is
sometimes subordinate to the opinion of a lay jury under the
(legal) direction of a judge; and compulsory psychiatric treatment (under English law anyway) is permitted (in most
circumstances) only at the instigation of a patient's relative or a
suitably qualified *non*-medical approved social worker. Such
dilutions of medical authority (which are fully endorsed by
most doctors) are partly a reflection of the fact that medical
opinion in cases of this sort is so diverse. They are also an
acknowledgement – tacit, to be sure – that there is more to
diagnostic opinion in such cases than merely the facts by which
the condition of a patient is defined, and to which, alone
perhaps, specifically medical testimony is truly expert. In just
what this "more" consists, we have no very clear idea. This is
one of the questions to which analytical research in medicine is

properly addressed. But it cannot be denied that opinion on illness-diagnostic questions, more so than opinion on condition-diagnostic questions, is at least influenced by such factors as the circumstances in which and the purposes for which a diagnosis is made. On the analogy of condition-diagnoses, this may perhaps be regretted. But it would not be right to regret it if the influence of such factors were in fact due to their being relevant.

Still, that is not the point to be argued here. The point for now is that if this somewhat painstaking approach to the problems with which we are here concerned has hinted at possible difficulties to come, these are really no more than the counterparts of difficulties which, on reflection, we know to be inherent in clinical work itself. At the very least, therefore, this correspondence shows the necessity in research of this kind, as in scientific research, of taking pains. Even, however, from the clinical point of view, it must now be clear that conceptual difficulties, if not actually to be welcomed, are also not to be avoided. If clinical work is difficult, and if it is difficult because, *inter alia*, it raises difficult conceptual questions, its requirements will be met, if at all, only by research in which these difficulties are met head on. Analytical research, therefore, if it is ever to contribute to better clinical practice, must be concerned to explicate, rather than side-step, clinical difficulties.

In the present work, then, our attitude to difficulties, be they clinical or analytical, is that they are our very meat. And once this attitude is established it reflects right through the assumptions with which we come to it. So far, assumption 2 in the conventional form of argument has only reluctantly been given up – namely, that 'physical illness', being unproblematic in clinical use, is an unproblematic concept. But now it is seen that if this were really so, if 'physical illness' really were an unproblematic concept, then there would be no good reason for clinical experience of the illness-diagnostic question (particularly, but not only, in psychological medicine) to be as problematic as it is. It might be supposed, unkindly, that doctors (particularly, but not only, in psychological medicine) are merely muddled; that the conceptual difficulties associated with illness-diagnostic questions are difficulties of their own making; that in respect of such difficulties, through ignorance, indifference or incapacity, they are simply failing to think straight. But what reason would there be for this? Why should doctors, more than others, be muddled? And why should doctors in psychological medicine be muddled more, and more often, than doctors in physical medicine? No, evidence of clinical difficulty is evidence only of just that, of clinical difficulty. Illness-diagnostic questions *are* difficult questions. And the concepts in which they are framed, not only 'mental illness' but also 'physical illness', *are* difficult concepts.

Corresponding changes are also required in our assumptions regarding 'mental illness'. Under assumption 1 in the conventional form of argument, it has been widely assumed that 'mental illness', being problematic clinically, is also problematic conceptually in any or all of the further three senses in which (under assumption 2) 'physical illness' is not – that is to say, as to perspicuity of definition, "soundness" and authenticity. But just as assumption 2 should now willingly, rather than reluctantly, be given up, because it stands in the way of progress, so, for the same reason, should assumption 1 now willingly be given up. Clinical difficulties are indeed associated with the use of the concept of 'mental illness' more than with that of 'physical illness'. But all that is shown by this observation is that 'mental illness' is the more difficult concept to work with clinically. There is nothing in the observation as such, to show that 'mental illness' is any less perspicuous, sound or authentic a concept than 'physical illness'. And to assume otherwise in a debate the very object of which is to establish the validity of the concept of 'mental illness' is more than a little tendentious.

Nor does the particular kind of clinical difficulty especially associated with 'mental illness', the illness-diagnostic difficulty, give grounds for assumption 1. For, as has been seen, illness-diagnostic difficulties, even amounting to contradictory diagnostic opinions, could actually be a faithful reflection of some property of the concept of 'illness'. In which case, mental illnesses (recalling sense 4 of assumption 2) would be at least as authentic examples of illnesses as are physical illnesses. Certainly, the particular features of 'mental illness' which render it more problematic diagnostically than 'physical illness' should not be thought of pejoratively. If 'mental illness', compared with 'physical illness', is – as Szasz and others of its opponents have emphasized – value-laden, subjective, vague in its connotations and variable in denotation, it is not thereby (recalling sense 3 of assumption 2) a defective concept. For these features of 'mental illness' could be, or could be products of, features of 'illness' itself. In which case, since these features are not so apparent in examples of physical illness, then 'mental illness' (recalling sense 2 of assumption 2), if not a wholly perspicuous concept, is here more, rather than less, perspicuous than 'physical illness'. Contrary to established practice, therefore, these features of 'mental illness' should be neither emphasized (as by its opponents) nor diminished or ignored (as by its supporters). They should rather be taken seriously in their own right, as features to be explained; and as features whose explanation could supply important lessons about the conceptual structure not only of psychological medicine but of medicine as a whole.

This is really the bottom line of this introductory chapter. By it, however, we are led to some final remarks on method – not on the form of argument to be pursued (which has already been set out), but on the method by which it is to be pursued. For in setting aside any preconceptions, pejorative or otherwise, about the concept of 'mental illness', and in recognizing that the concept of 'physical illness', contrary to clinical appearances, is conceptually at least as problematic as the concept of 'mental illness', we are brought to a definite conclusion about the way in which philosophy is most likely to be gainfully employed in resolving the conceptual difficulties associated with 'mental illness' in clinical use.

Thus, as long as the concept of 'mental illness' is thought to be *the* problem with which we are concerned (as under assumption 1), and as long as the concept of 'physical illness' is thought *not* to be a problem (as under assumption 2), it is natural that we should turn for enlightenment to those branches of general philosophy that bear most directly on the differences between these two concepts. First, and most obviously perhaps, if it is the "mental" in 'mental illness' which is thought to be at fault, we might turn to the philosophy of mind; or, since psychological medicine is less well developed (because it is more difficult) scientifically than physical medicine, to the philosophy of science. Indeed, both these, as well as other branches of philosophy, have been drawn on in the debate about 'mental illness': see, for instance, Roth and Kroll (1986, Ch. 4) for the mind–body problem; and Slater (1973) and Bebbington (1977) for the philosophy of science. Then again, the nominalist–essentialist debate has figured prominently in discussions especially of disease concepts – the issues are thoroughly discussed by Rezneck (1987), for example; and Gillon (1986), amongst others, has pointed out the interesting conceptual connections between this debate and the question with which this book is concerned, namely, whether the medical concepts are value-free. It is true, of course, that the nature of the problems with which general philosophy is occupied is such that ready-made solutions to clinical problems are unlikely to be derived directly from it, by philosophical short-cuts, as it were. But once it is recognized that it is the concepts employed in medicine generally with which we are concerned, rather than just those employed in psychological medicine, even the motive for such short-cut taking disappears. For it is then clear that, in advance of an analysis of these concepts, we can have no reliable idea, even, in just what the clinically problematic nature of 'mental illness' consists. So that in default of such an analysis, we can have no reliable idea which branch or branches of general philosophy might be helpful to us, even in principle. Before turning to general philosophy, therefore, a straightforward conceptual analysis of medicine is required.

But, it may be objected, general philosophy, or much of philosophy in the Anglo-Saxon tradition at least, is occupied with the analysis of concepts. Indeed, one branch of philosophy is marked off from another mainly by the concepts with which it is specifically concerned. And if the foregoing is just a plea for a branch of philosophy specially concerned with the concepts employed in medicine, it should not be forgotten that different philosophical disciplines, like different medical disciplines, are strongly interdependent. The philosopher of mind, say, can no more afford to be ignorant of epistemology or the philosophy of action or the free-will problem than an ophthalmologist can afford to be ignorant of hypertension, diabetes or general neurology. A degree of specialization is inevitable. All the more so in philosophies of disciplines such as medicine, to which so much practical knowledge and experience are pertinent. But philosophers of medicine, like those of physics, law, sociology and the rest, though perhaps not primarily concerned with the problems of general philosophy, are certainly not isolated from them.

The relationship between philosophy and medicine will be considered in more detail and in the light of the findings in this book in the concluding chapter. But there is nothing in the views expressed in the preceding paragraph with which we should disagree. Indeed, the method by which the present analysis is to be pursued is one which is borrowed from general philosophy – namely, the method of linguistic analysis. This method, which is based on a view of the nature of philosophical problems put forward by the Austrian-born Cambridge philosopher Ludwig Wittgenstein, in the period between the two world wars, is described, for example, by Austin (1956–7). It is not a well-defined technique like the techniques, say, of cardiac surgery or of passing a driving test. Rather, like the scientific method, it is a way of tackling problems of a particular kind, obvious enough in principle, yet sometimes having uncommon problem-solving power if pursued with determination and rigour. The analogy should certainly not be pressed too far. But where science is concerned with facts, philosophy is concerned with concepts; where the scientific method for discerning facts is based on careful, comprehensive observations of empirical data, linguistic analysis, as a philosophical method, is based on careful, comprehensive observations of linguistic data (including the ways in which and the purposes for which concepts are actually employed in any given real-life situation or area of discourse); and where in the case of the scientific method it is possible to go beyond common sense by testing the facts as they are assumed to be against empirical data, so in the case of the method of linguistic analysis it is possible to go beyond common sense by testing concepts as they are assumed to be against linguistic data, against what people actually say.

The idea is simple enough. A conceptual difficulty, it is supposed, whether in philosophy as such or in some other discipline such as clinical medicine, may arise from an excessive preoccupation with some particular aspect or feature of the concept in question. A conceptual difficulty of this kind thus either is, or is the result of, a distorted view of that concept. But our concepts are reflected in the things we say. Therefore it should be possible to correct the distortions in our view of that concept, and thus to resolve the difficulties resulting from them, by looking carefully and comprehensively at whatever is said in terms of it. The trick, however, as in science, is to make the pertinent observations. For if the difficulties are of this kind – if they are the result, essentially, of illusions – no small effort of imagination may be required to escape from them. By the very nature of the problem, whatever is obvious or familiar or commonplace is to be mistrusted. As Hare (1978) has remarked, what is required for analytical work of this kind is good peripheral vision.

It follows, therefore, that in setting aside at least for the moment the deep questions of general philosophy, in confining ourselves initially to the more prosaic task of analysing the language of medicine, we are left with no lightweight undertaking. The objective so defined is no less than a comprehensive explanation of ordinary medical usage, in non-technical as well as in technical contexts, in physical as well as in psychological medicine, in general practice and in other areas of primary health care as well as in hospital practice, and among nurses, psychologists, social workers, lawyers and administrators, as well as among doctors. Granted this way of understanding the nature of philosophical enquiry, the extent to which this objective is achieved by the present or any other view of the conceptual structure of medicine is a criterion of the success of that view. This is a pre-set outcome criterion, as it were. This criterion encompasses, without being limited to, the more familiar criteria of validity in philosophy; that is, besides imaginative open-mindedness and an alert eye, internal consistency and close attention to the rules of formal logic. This criterion, furthermore, is supplemented in the present case by the two requirements noted earlier, arising from the form of the debate about mental illness; a requirement that the analysis must show whether there is a general concept 'illness' distinct from 'physical illness', and a requirement that it show reasons both for the similarities and the differences between 'physical illness' and 'mental illness' in ordinary usage. We may hope that the analysis will show much else besides. But this much at least it must show if we are to be able to proceed with any confidence to a consideration of the difficulties which first gave rise to the mental-illness debate, the conceptual difficulties raised by "mental illness" in clinical practice.

Yet it is with precisely these clinical difficulties that we are ultimately concerned. Lest, therefore, anyone imagine that the results of analytical research of the kind to be pursued here are likely to be somewhat remote from the contingencies of everyday clinical work, it should finally be said that it is by just these clinical contingencies that in the present case a second and more acid outcome criterion is supplied. There will be more to say about this later. But it can at any rate be seen that, however well our results stand up under the first outcome criterion, however comprehensively they explain ordinary medical usage, they can hardly be considered complete unless they make at least some contribution to resolving the conceptual difficulties in clinical practice from which the very need for conceptual analysis in medicine has arisen.

ILLNESS AND DISEASE
AS VALUE TERMS

Part II

2

The conventional view

In ordinary usage, 'illness' is closely identified with 'disease', which in turn is closely identified with 'dysfunction'. In the Shorter Oxford English Dictionary, for example, the word 'disease' appears in the definition of 'illness', and vice versa. Moreover, 'disease', though not 'illness', is further defined in terms of 'dysfunction' as "a condition of the body, or of some part or organ of the body, in which its functions are disturbed or deranged".

These features of everyday usage have often been carried over, sometimes more, sometimes less overtly, into the literature. A distinction between 'illness' and 'disease' has been recognized (for example Barondess, 1979). But in much of the debate about 'mental illness', 'disease' and 'illness' have been not merely identified with each other, but treated as synonyms. And the meaning of this combined concept 'illness/disease', has then been analysed, essentially along the lines of the Shorter Oxford English Dictionary definition of 'disease', in terms of disturbance of function of one kind or another. This approach is adopted, for example, by both Kendell and Szasz, whose views, respectively for and against the concept of 'mental illness', were noted in the last chapter. Both these authors use 'illness' and 'disease' as synonyms; and both interpret the meaning of 'illness/disease' in terms of 'dysfunction' – albeit differently defined, and crucially so, their different definitions leading to different conclusions about 'mental illness'.

Yet the three terms 'illness', 'disease' and 'dysfunction', although closely related in meaning (being used, for example, in similar contexts, of similar conditions, and with similar implications), are none the less not always logically interchangeable. Sometimes, it is true, 'disease' may properly be used as a synonym for 'illness'; "He has some awful illness", for example, would normally mean the same as "He has some awful disease." Similarly, 'disease' may sometimes properly be used as a synonym for 'dysfunction'; the term 'obstructive airways disease' means essentially a disturbance of lung function with a characteristic impairment of airflow. Further, a great many individual diseases, especially in physical medicine, are defined by specific impairments of this or that bodily function. But against instances such as these, there are clear cases in which 'disease' and 'illness', at least, are used not only with different but with contrasting meanings. Thus a diabetic whose condition is fully controlled by treatment would properly be said to have the disease diabetes, but not to be ill; and a patient with an asymptomatic cancer detected coincidentally, in the course of a life insurance examination say, could be spoken of in much the same way. Then again, while many disease categories are indeed defined in terms of impairments of bodily function, many others, such as migraine, are not. To say that someone has migraine is to say just that they are suffering or sometimes suffer a particular kind of headache (one-sided, relapsing and so on). Headaches of this kind (it would nowadays normally be assumed) may turn out to be *caused* by some (as yet undiscovered) disturbance of bodily function. Similarly, they may *cause* the sufferer to function less than optimally. But migraine none the less does not consist in – it is not *defined by* – disturbance of function.

All this is of course not to say that 'illness', 'disease' and 'dysfunction' cannot be defined, by one route or another, in terms of each other. On the contrary, their *prima-facie* close relationship in ordinary (that is, both colloquial and technical) usage, together with their actual use in certain contexts as synonyms, makes this at least likely; though it is part of the purpose of this book to suggest that the key to understanding the relationship between them is a fourth concept, introduced first in chapter 7 under the name 'action failure'. But the point for now is simply that *any* account of the relationship between 'illness', 'disease' and 'dysfunction' must address not only the synonymous but also the non-synonymous uses of these concepts.

This point has been taken by a number of authors in the literature on the medical concepts. Boorse, in particular, in his paper "On the distinction between illness and disease" (1975), makes it central. He argues thus. At the heart of many of the issues with which medicine has become involved recently – sexual deviation, criminal responsibility and so on – is a "fundamental misunderstanding of the concept of 'health' ", namely, that it is an "evaluative notion" (p. 49). This misunderstanding arises from a confusion between the "theoretical" and "practical" senses of 'health', or, in terms of their opposites, between 'disease' and 'illness'. Boorse then analyses the distinction between 'disease' and 'illness' as a distinction between a factual term and a value term. 'Disease', he says, although sometimes used colloquially as a synonym for 'illness', is in "technical usage" – that is, "as found in textbooks of medical theory" (p. 50) – analysable in terms of 'dysfunction'; hence, since 'dysfunction' is "continuous with theory in biology and the other natural sciences, 'disease' is value free" (p. 55). 'Illness', on the other hand, is an evaluative notion. Illnesses are "merely a subclass of disease" consisting of those diseases which (as in the cases of diabetes and cancer noted above) are "reasonably serious", and hence "incapacitating"; and it is from this that their evaluative features – that they are "undesirable" and so on – are derived. Boorse thus concludes that to say someone is ill is indeed to express a value judgement. But since it is 'disease', as used in medical theory, which is the more fundamental concept, and since in this use 'disease' is value-free, so too, and fundamentally, is the concept of 'health'.

In the next chapter we will be looking in detail at the claim which is at the heart of Boorse's analysis, and indeed at the heart of all so-called "medical" models, namely that 'dysfunction', at least as used in technical contexts in medicine, is value-free. For the moment, though, we should note, first, the wide range of features of ordinary usage that are fully consistent with his views. 'Illness', as well as 'disease' used as a synonym for 'illness', certainly is found in non-technical more than in technical contexts. Moreover, it does have clear evaluative connotations. It is used by patients or their relatives, for example to complain, to say that "something is *wrong*", to express or evoke concern, to provoke a therapeutic response. (It is this feature of 'illness', by the way, which lies behind apparently tautological definitions of the medical concepts in terms of their ability to "arouse therapeutic concern", e.g., Taylor, 1983.) Further, as with other value terms, there is wide variation, both individual and cultural, in the conditions in respect of which 'illness' is used. Though since these conditions are usually defined in terms of subjective sensations – that is, in terms of the very symptoms of illness, pain, dizziness and the like – they are, more so even than many other value terms, often peculiarly ill-defined and unreliably reported and described. 'Disease', however, as a term distinct in meaning from 'illness', is used more in technical contexts. It is used by doctors rather than by patients or their relatives. It is used to express *what* is wrong, to describe, by way of clearly defined objective bodily changes in so far as it is possible, the condition from which a patient is suffering, and thus to identify that condition with one or more of the categories in some mutually agreed classification of diseases. Furthermore, although many such classifications are possible in principle, those employed in practice are those which best serve the purposes for which a diagnosis is being made. For medical purposes, which include curing or alleviating illness, though not always for other purposes – for example, administrative or legal purposes, as in respect of mental deficiency – the most useful classifications are those based on causes. The causes of illness, even bodily causes, are protean: infections, intoxications, inflammations and so on. But the common factor, the final common causal pathway, is often, as Boorse himself indicates, some disturbance of function. Historically, therefore, as knowledge of the causes of illness becomes available from the results of scientific research, disease categories defined in terms of symptoms (such as migraine) become displaced by categories defined in terms of causes, with disturbances of bodily function becoming increasingly prominent. And this evolution is then recapitulated, albeit in an abbreviated form, each time an individual diagnosis is made. Thus, all in all, as Wing puts it (1978, p. 23) most "well-developed" disease theories are now drawn, as Boorse maintains they should be drawn, in terms of disturbances of bodily function.

Boorse's analysis of the relationships between 'illness', 'disease' and 'dysfunction' thus incorporates, and so is consistent with, many important properties of these concepts in ordinary usage. Yet there are other properties of these concepts with which Boorse's analysis is on the face of it wholly *in*consistent. How, for example, could his theory explain instances in which someone may be said to be ill without being said to have a disease, as in the case of a hangover, say, or following an overdose? Boorse's theory, that 'illness' is a *subcategory* of 'disease', explains cases (for example, our diabetic/cancer cases above) in which one may be said to have a disease but not to be ill; but the same subcategory theory cannot also explain contrary cases, of the hangover type. We will see later (chapters 4, 5 and 8), that cases of this kind are in an important sense marginal; for example, one might want to say of someone with a hangover – though perhaps not following an overdose – that they only feel ill. To this extent, then, it may be thought that cases of this kind are not too damaging to Boorse's account (though the "marginal" status of such cases has still to be explained; see, in the present account, chapters 5 and 7 in particular). But Boorse's subcategory theory of illness also cannot explain the more common case in which a patient may be said to be ill even though the particular (Boorse-type) disease – that is, the particular disturbance of function – from which he is suffering has not yet been diagnosed. Then again, Boorse's subcategory theory of 'illness' runs into difficulties with regard to the particular evaluative features by which his illness-subcategory is taken to be defined. One such feature is that 'disease', but not 'illness', is used as readily of plants and animals as of people. This, Boorse says, is because of differences in the kinds of value judgement we are prepared to make about people and other living things. In this he may well be right; certainly there *are* such differences. But Boorse's theory of 'illness' is that its evaluative features – that it is undesirable and so on – are derived from its being a disease which is "serious enough to be incapacitating" (1975, p. 61). However, if this were really so, if the relationship between 'illness' and 'disease' were really as simple as this, then we should be as ready to say that a disease-incapacitated plant or animal is ill as that a disease-incapacitated person is ill. But we are not.

Still more substantial difficulties for Boorse's analysis are presented by 'dysfunction' in its (logical) relationships both with 'disease' and with 'illness'. Thus, with regard to 'disease', Boorse's theory requires that all diseases, properly speaking, be disturbances of function. But this is simply not so. Neither are all disturbances of function, even of bodily function, diseases. Diseases are only one species of "malady" (Culver and Gert's generic term, 1982). Other dysfunctional conditions are wounds, for example; others are congenital or some kinds of chronic disability. Definitions of 'disease' of the Boorse- and, indeed, the dictionary-variety, which simply reduce it to 'dysfunction' – and a large majority of so-called medical models are of this kind – are therefore, in Flew's phrase, altogether too "broad" (1973, p. 35). If such definitions are to be satisfactory, at least some account of the particular kinds of dysfunction by which 'disease' is defined must be given. Then again, as to the relationship between 'dysfunction' and 'illness', this would seem to be entirely different in ordinary usage from that suggested by Boorse. For Boorse's theory is that 'illness' is a subcategory of 'disease' which in turn equals 'disturbance of function'. But if this is right, then to say that someone is ill is to say that they are not functioning properly. Yet this is not how we ordinarily speak. Ordinarily, it is *people* who fall ill, and their *bodies* (or parts or organs thereof) which, in the required sense, fail to function properly. Substitute 'not functioning properly' in a statement such as 'he is ill', and you get something quite different from the original. The expression 'He is not functioning properly', if used at all, would ordinarily be taken to mean not that the person in question is ill, but that he is not functioning properly in some social role, as a parent, or a footballer, say. The relationship between 'dysfunction' and 'illness' is thus, at the very least, more subtle than Boorse suggests. And this conclusion is underlined by the fact noted earlier in this chapter that despite their logical non-equivalence, 'dysfunction' and 'illness' are connected by a logical bridge, a bridge of meaning, which is formed by 'disease'

32

having the capacity in different contexts to be synonymous with either.

These difficulties might be thought to be less damaging to Boorse's analysis if it is understood not as failing to explain certain aspects of ordinary usage, but rather as concentrating on those particular aspects which are important for the purposes of medical theory. Boorse's strategy, after all, is based on the idea that if 'disease', defined value-free in terms of the biological-scientific facts of disturbed functioning, is prominent in technical contexts in medicine, then this is for the good reason that, so defined, it has in the past proved so effective in respect of the problems with which doctors are concerned. So defined, indeed, 'disease' corresponds with the medical model by means of which medicine as a scientific discipline has made such rapid progress in recent times. Under the first outcome criterion appropriate to analytical research, therefore, that of explaining ordinary usage, there may be deficiencies in Boorse's analysis. But it is under the second outcome criterion, that of practical utility, that it may be thought to be more appropriately judged.

The past success of the medical model, however, is really a most insecure basis from which to defend its use in the context of analytical research. This is because this success has been in respect of *empirical* clinical problems – indeed, the model is really a medical-scientific model – whereas the problems with which analytical research in medicine is concerned are primarily *non*-empirical. There is no antagonism here, of course. Any satisfactory account of the conceptual structure of medicine must successfully incorporate medical science. But there can be no guaranteed transfer of success from empirical to non-empirical areas of research. On the contrary, for, as noted in chapter 1, the growth in recent years of non-empirical problems in medicine, is, in part, a direct result of medical-scientific progress. Thus to adopt for analytical research purposes a medical-scientific model could well be to compound the very problems which such research seeks to address. There is in fact evidence of this in the applied part of Boorse's paper. His treatment of 'homosexuality', for example, far from clarifying what he calls the "disputatious" disease status of this condition, in effect merely redefines the scope of medical theory so as to exclude the dispute. And the main thrust of his argument is after all in this way proscriptive. He seeks generally to exclude the logical element of evaluation from medical theory. But this is to do no more than to duplicate in analysis the burgeoning of science in medicine. It follows, therefore, that to the extent that Boorse's theory fails to account for the logical properties of the medical concepts, this could be because these concepts – not just 'illness', but also 'disease' and even 'dysfunction' – are not, at bottom, value-free at all.

3

Dysfunction

The question raised at the end of the last chapter, whether the terms 'disease' and 'dysfunction' are really value-free as used in technical contexts in medicine, is an important question. It is central not only to Boorse's view of the medical concepts but to "medical" models generally. That it should be raised at all, however, is due to a property which 'disease' and 'dysfunction' have in common with 'illness' – namely, that although etymologically value terms, and although capable of being used as such, they may also be used (as in technical contexts in medicine) with mainly factual rather than evaluative connotations. This property has in fact been important in the debate about 'mental illness'. As we saw in chapter 1, Szasz-type objections to 'mental illness' gain credibility from the fact that all three terms, 'dysfunction' and 'disease' as well as 'illness', tend to have more marked evaluative connotations when they are used in respect of mental, as opposed to physical, conditions. While the basis of Kendell-type replies to such objections is that, none the less, the factual content of all three terms is essentially the same. Boorse's (reconciling) theory, on the other hand, stems from the observation that in respect of either kind of condition, mental or physical, 'illness' has by and large the most, and 'dysfunction' the least, marked evaluative connotations of the three.

This double-aspect property as to fact and value is, however, not unique to the medical terms. On the contrary, it is a property shared by a great many terms, and certainly by all value terms. Hare (1963a) and others have noted that even those most generic of value terms, 'good' and 'bad', often convey, as part of their meaning, definite factual information; so that the relevant distinction in this context is perhaps not between value terms and factual terms as such, but rather

35

between the evaluative and factual *uses* of a given term. Furthermore, just as this property as a property of medical value terms has been important in medicine in the debate about 'mental illness', so, as a property of value terms in general it has been important in ethics, in the so-called "is–ought" debate. Indeed, the question raised at the end of the last chapter can be understood as a special case of a more general question at the heart of the is–ought debate. The question here is whether the medical terms 'disease' and 'dysfunction', though etymologically value terms, are value-free as used in technical contexts in medicine. The more general question is whether *any* value term may *ever* be used in this way – that is to say, whether any expression of value (including 'ought') may ever be defined purely descriptively (in terms of 'is').

The is–ought debate is still unresolved. For some, indeed, the debate itself is ill-founded; it has been claimed, from a variety of philosophical points of view, that there is really no such thing as a value-free fact to which we can go on to attach value (for example, Melden, 1959; Winch, 1972; McDowell, 1978; Williams, 1985). Among those for whom the debate is well-founded, however, recent philosophical opinion has perhaps swung somewhat against the "descriptivist" view that (as required by "medical" models) at least *some* value terms may at least in *some* uses be defined descriptively. The alternative, "non-descriptivist" view has gained ground: the view, first set out clearly by the eighteenth-century empiricist philosopher David Hume in Book III of his Treatise, that there is a logical divide between facts and values; that to get an 'ought' out of the meaning of an expression, so to speak, an 'ought' has first to be put in; and hence that expressions of value may *never* be analysed into, or defined in terms of, statements of fact alone. But whatever the final outcome of this deabte, the arguments and counter-arguments of the two sides, descriptivist and non-descriptivist, are highly instructive when applied to the specifically medical question with which we are concerned here.

The remainder of this chapter, then, will be taken up with an examination of some of these arguments and counter-arguments. The discussion will be dramatized in the form of a debate about Boorse's version of the medical model (as described generally in chapter 2) between two imaginary philosophers, one broadly descriptivist in outlook, the other broadly non-descriptivist. As we will see, the views of these two philosophers run a long way parallel. There is a good deal about which they agree. But it is their point of disagreement – on the is–ought divide – that is crucial to the analysis of the medical concepts set out in this book.

The debate

NON-DESCRIPTIVIST: On the face of it, Boorse's views, strictly interpreted, are surely rather implausible . . .

If it is true, as he claims, that 'dysfunction' and 'disease' are (in technical contexts in medicine) purely descriptive terms, why is it that he repeatedly slips into using them evaluatively? In his 1975 paper, for example, he first defines 'disease' descriptively as ". . . a deviation from the natural (= statistically typical) functional organisation of the species . . . " (p. 59). But by the second time around, only two lines later, 'disease' has become "a deficiency in the functional efficiency of the body". The descriptive 'deviant functional organisation' has become the evaluative 'deficient functional efficiency'.

DESCRIPTIVIST: I agree. Boorse's *claim* notwithstanding, he continues to use both 'dysfunction' and 'disease', and the ideas expressed by these terms, evaluatively.

There really is no value judgement involved in the claim that the functional organization of an organism deviates in some respect from that which is typical of the species to which it belongs; after all, its deviant functional organization might be better or worse or of equal merit. But the claim that it is functionally inefficient clearly does involve a value judgement of some kind – that it is not functioning *well*, for example, or *properly* or *successfully* or as it *ought* to function.

NON-DESCRIPTIVIST: We do not have to look far for a

37

second example. In the same section of Boorse's paper we find the term 'hostile' used evaluatively.

This occurs at the point at which Boorse seeks to extend his definition of 'disease' to cover conditions such as tooth decay which, although diseases, are statistically *typical* conditions. In order to encompass such conditions, Boorse broadens his definition of 'deviation from the natural' to include not only statistically atypical conditions, but also those "mainly due to environmental causes". But once again, the second time around – in this case three lines later – the descriptive 'environmental causes' becomes the evaluative '*hostile* environment'.

DESCRIPTIVIST: The most obvious examples of this slipping from fact to value occur later on in Boorse's 1975 paper, and again in a 1976 paper, when he deals with mental conditions.

Thus, in the 1975 paper (p. 62) he defines 'mental disease' (ostensibly on his value-free model of physical disease) as an "*interference*" with a mental function. But what is there to distinguish an interference from an enhancement, other than a value judgement? If Boorse meant to be evaluatively neutral here – that is, if his intended meaning did not include a value judgement – then why did he not use an evaluatively neutral term such as 'effect'?

That his definition of 'mental disease' is in fact not evaluatively neutral is clear from what he goes on to say (in both papers) about particular mental diseases. In the 1975 paper (p. 65) he claims that neuroses are mental diseases (according to his definition) because they can be "*blamed*" on an "*injurious*" cultural environment, which fills children's minds with "*excessive* anxieties", "*grotesque* role models" and "*absurd* prejudices". And in the 1976 paper he says that at least some psychoses are diseases because they lead to "biologically *incompetent* behaviour" (p. 76) and/or "*disrupted* . . . cognitive functions" (p. 77).

One such value judgement might be a slip of the pen. But they appear time and time again.

NON-DESCRIPTIVIST: Of course, Boorse does allow value

judgements by ordinary, rather than by strict, implication; that is to say, value judgements that are implied by virtue of the fact that to have a disease is to be in a condition which generally *is* negatively evaluated, rather than by virtue of there being a negative value judgement built into the very *meaning* of the term 'disease', let alone that of 'dysfunction'.

DESCRIPTIVIST: Yes, but this is not how value judgements are slipping in here.

Boorse's own example of ordinary implication, the positive value judgement which is often implied by the descriptive term 'intelligent', helps to establish this point.

Thus, he notes that intelligence is a quality which tends to be evaluated positively (1975, p. 55). Hence describing someone as intelligent tends to carry positive evaluative connotations; and this is particularly so when we are speaking loosely, in everyday, non-technical contexts. But, Boorse continues, the term 'intelligent' is none the less a purely descriptive term. Its exact descriptive meaning is somewhat complicated, no doubt, and its meaning may even vary to some extent from one context to another (for example, from one psychology textbook to another). But notwithstanding these complications and variations, its meaning is purely descriptive all the same. And in technical contexts, when we are using the term carefully, this is how it is used, *as* a purely descriptive term.

NON-DESCRIPTIVIST: Thus far we can agree with Boorse.

DESCRIPTIVIST: Certainly. But now consider 'disease' and 'dysfunction'. Are these terms like 'intelligent' in the required respects, as Boorse suggests?

Well, there are similarities, certainly. In the first place, being diseased, or not functioning properly, are conditions which generally are evaluated (in this case) negatively. Moreover, the terms 'disease' and 'dysfunction' clearly carry, as an important part of their meaning, descriptive information – albeit information like that carried by the term 'intelligent', which is not only complex but varies with context.

But there, and crucially, the similarities end. For when we are speaking carefully in technical contexts (as Boorse himself is speaking in his two papers), 'disease' and 'dysfunction', unlike 'intelligent', continue to be used (as by Boorse himself) evaluatively. And this is just what we would expect if value judgements are indeed part of the very meanings of these terms. If this is so, however, then it is obviously not possible – indeed, it is *strictly* impossible – for these terms to be used without implying a value judgement. The value judgement may not be obvious or overt; but if it is part of the *meaning* of these terms, it will necessarily be there.

NON-DESCRIPTIVIST: Yes, I agree.

DESCRIPTIVIST: But what I should now like to suggest is that perhaps we are being unfair to Boorse in interpreting his model so literally.

Perhaps we should reinterpret it as resting not on the possibly over-simple idea that 'disease' and 'dysfunction', as used in medicine, are purely descriptive terms (though this is indeed what Boorse seems to believe), but rather on the idea that although these terms *are* value terms, the value judgements expressed by them are *entailed by* certain descriptions.

NON-DESCRIPTIVIST: We are coming to the crunch!

DESCRIPTIVIST: No doubt! But let's look at this suggestion . . .

Boorse's claim, as we have interpreted it so far, is that to say of an organism that it has a disease or that it is not functioning properly, is *simply* to describe it in certain ways. Perhaps, as he suggests in his 1975 paper (p. 57), and as many others have suggested, it is to describe its functional state as one which consists or results in reduced life and/or reproductive expectations.

But reinterpreted in the way I am now suggesting, Boorse's claim becomes the rather more complicated claim that the value judgements expressed by the terms 'disease' and 'dysfunction' are entailed by this same description. And this is a much more plausible claim, I believe.

NON-DESCRIPTIVIST: This is where we part company, then, for your reinterpretation of Boorse's claim is along descriptivist lines not unlike those adopted by Philippa Foot (1958/9), for example, in her analysis of 'dangerous'.

DESCRIPTIVIST: Possibly so. But descriptivism is distinctly attractive here, since it offers Boorse (and the authors of other similar medical models) the best of two worlds.

On the one hand, it resolves the conflict just noted between descriptive analyses of the terms 'disease' and 'dysfunction', and the continued use of these terms as value terms. For if the value judgements expressed by 'disease' and 'dysfunction' are entailed by certain descriptions (such as those into which they are analysed by Boorse), then the two kinds of expression, value judgement and description, are entirely consistent with one another.

On the other hand, descriptivism gives Boorse what he is really after, or as much of what he is after as his own analysis gives him – namely, as he puts it, "a value free science of health" (1975, p. 49). For if 'dysfunction' and 'disease', although value terms, are entailed by certain de-scriptions, then it will always be possible – at least to the extent of this entailment – to translate the value judgements expressed by them back into these descriptions. Boorse's claim, interpreted literally, would, if correct, provide for a value-free science of health to the extent that 'dysfunction' and 'disease' are purely descriptive terms. But his claim, reinterpreted as a descriptivist claim, also provides for a value-free science of health to the extent that the value judgements expressed by 'dysfunction' and 'disease' may be translated back into (because they are entailed by) purely descriptive terms.

NON-DESCRIPTIVIST: I suppose one objection, from a medical point of view, to reinterpreting Boorse's claims in this way, is that it seems to turn a relatively straightforward thesis – one rather easy to understand – into something that appears philosophically convoluted.

DESCRIPTIVIST: Yes, but this is a matter for Occam's razor – if the simpler thesis fits, fine: if not, we have to go for something more complicated.

In fact, though, if there is a difficulty here, if the descriptivist reinterpretation of Boorse's claim appears convoluted, this is not so much because it is complicated as because it is just unfamiliar.

NON-DESCRIPTIVIST: And besides, if I could make a point in support of descriptivism, there is an important sense in which your descriptivist reinterpretation of Boorse's claim is actually simpler than the original – that is, in that rather less is required to sustain it. And for this reason, at least, it "fits", as you put it, better than the original.

DESCRIPTIVIST: Certainly, and that is a point in support of my suggestion that this is how Boorse's theory should be understood.

Let me spell the point out ... the minimum requirement, all that is necessary to sustain Boorse's claim, reinterpreted as a descriptivist claim, is simply this: that in evaluating the functional state of an organism, *if* we are prepared to describe its functional state as one which consists or results in reduced life and/or reproductive expectations, *then*, by virtue only of the meanings of the terms 'dysfunction' and 'disease', we are obliged to evaluate its functional state negatively, *as* a dysfunctional state, and the organism itself *as* diseased.

This is all that is required. The converse is not required. There is no requirement that in taking an organism to have a disease or to be dysfunctioning we should take its functional state to be one which consists or results in reduced life and/or reproductive expectations. Hence, as against the original, this reinterpreted version of Boorse's claim is not invalidated by the fact that many diseases – for example, migraine – are wholly *un*related to functional states consisting or resulting in reduced life and/or reproductive expectations. Furthermore, the reinterpreted claim does not require that there be no *other* descriptions by which 'dysfunction' and 'disease' are entailed. Indeed, there may well be such, and clarification of these other descriptions would then be an important task for analytical research in medicine.

So, provided the minimum requirement is satisfied, I believe we have, in the description "functional state consisting or resulting in reduced life and/or reproductive expectations", at least the beginnings of sound descriptivist analyses of 'dysfunction' and 'disease'.

NON-DESCRIPTIVIST: Well, that is what we have to test.

But shall we agree, now, to simplify the remainder of our discussion by confining ourselves to 'dysfunction' and leaving aside 'disease'? The question with which we are concerned is the same for both terms: namely, are they capable of being analysed descriptively, even though they are value terms? In answering this question, however, 'dysfunction' is the more important for us to concentrate on. For, having less marked evaluative connotations than 'disease', it is the more likely candidate for, and hence provides a better test case of, descriptivist analysis. Presumably it is for this same reason that Boorse's model, and other similar models, are based on 'dysfunction' rather than 'disease'. Hence, in concentrating on 'dysfunction', our conclusions will automatically go straight to the foundations of medical models of this kind.

DESCRIPTIVIST: I would go along with that.

However, we should add an important proviso. In agreeing to simplify our discussion in this way, we should not be committed to the idea that 'dysfunction' necessarily occupies any special or central conceptual place in medicine. It may do so. And in most medical models it is assumed that it does. In Boorse's model, for example, 'disease' is in effect treated merely as a *sub*category of 'dysfunction'. But if 'disease' *is* a subcategory of 'dysfunction', it is not the subcategory suggested by Boorse: for a dysfunctional state which is due to the influence of a "hostile environment" would be a wound or an injury, surely, not a disease, while the evaluatively neutral "environmental-causes" version of this would preclude endemic genetic diseases.

NON-DESCRIPTIVIST: I agree with the proviso and would like to add that this problem with Boorse's theory could well be a symptom of some more serious underlying defect in the foundations of his model. Specifically, it could be a sign that 'dysfunction' is not value-free.

Furthermore, and conversely, if in our present discussion we now conclude that 'dysfunction' as used in medicine is *not* value-free, we might reasonably take this as sufficient justification for questioning whether 'dysfunction' is conceptually central in medicine at all. At the very least, if 'dysfunction' is not value-free, or at any rate capable of value-free definition, much of the motivation for *making* it conceptually central in medicine disappears. And the way is then clear for alternative models to be considered: models in which neither 'disease' nor 'dysfunction' is conceptually central, but rather the more overtly evaluative concept 'illness'; and in which the relationships between all three concepts may perhaps be more satisfactorily derived than in Boorse's model, from their properties *as* value terms (see chapter 4).

DESCRIPTIVIST: Still, all this is clearly beyond the scope of our present discussion.

NON-DESCRIPTIVIST: Agreed. But to come back to 'dysfunction', the crunch point between us is, can the use of this term in technical contexts in medicine (whether conceptually central or not) be analysed, as required by Boorse's and other medical models, in purely factual, value-free terms.

Your view, that it may be so analysed, is, as I have already said, a standardly descriptivist view. As such, there are a number of standard non-descriptivist objections to it. But before going into these, there is an obvious objection to Boorse's particular version of this view, surely, in that its "minimum requirement", as we called it earlier, is not in fact satisfied. For, contrary to this requirement, there *are* functional states of organisms which, although they would (ordinarily) be described as states consisting or resulting in reduced life and/or reproductive expectations, none the less would *not* (ordinarily) be evaluated as dysfunctional states, let alone diseases – the functional state of racing-car driving, for example.

DESCRIPTIVIST: I am willing to concede that objection, at least in principle, though, as I will argue in a moment, I think that rather little is lost to descriptivism thereby.

However, just to get the objection clear, what would you say to the counter-objection against your example of racing-car driving that the concept of 'function' is one which is applicable more to the parts of an organism – to its organs, limbs, physiological systems and so on – than to the organism as a whole?

NON-DESCRIPTIVIST: Just that while it is true that we do not speak, for example, of *the* function of a man (in the way that we speak of *the* function of a kidney, say), we do speak of men having functions and of men functioning (*as* racing-car drivers, *as* parents and so forth), which is all that is required for my example.

DESCRIPTIVIST: Yes, I agree with that.

Then there is a related counter-objection, that your example of racing-car driving bites on Boorse's definition mainly as applied to social functioning, which is *prima facie* somewhat further (conceptually) than bodily functioning from 'disease'. What would your reply be to that?

NON-DESCRIPTIVIST: First, that I would agree with the counter-objection to the extent that the relationship between 'social functioning' and 'disease' is more problematic than that between 'bodily functioning' and 'disease'.

But against this, any actual *proscription* of social functioning from the definition of disease (as proposed by Boorse in terms of disturbed functioning) would make a number at least of mental illnesses, in Szasz's terms, "mythological". Childhood autism, for example, and to an important extent schizophrenia, consist in impaired social functioning. And Boorse's purpose, surely, far from being to exclude conditions such as these, is to put 'mental disease' on the same conceptual footing as 'physical disease'.

My main point stands, therefore. Boorse's criteria of reduced life and/or reproductive expectations, fails even as a minimum criterion of impaired functioning. Contrary to what we said earlier, it is *not* true that if one is prepared to describe the functional state of an organism as consisting or resulting in reduced life and/or reproductive expectations, then by virtue only of the meaning of 'dysfunction' one is obliged to evaluate its functional state negatively, *as* a dysfunctional state (and the same is true, of course, *mutatis mutandis*, for 'disease').

DESCRIPTIVIST: Again, I agree.

Let me then take up the point I anticipated a moment ago. Granted your objection to Boorse's definition, how much is lost to descriptivism thereby?

So far as Boorse's particular theory is concerned, your objection shows, certainly, that his definition of 'dysfunction' should be restricted in application, perhaps to bodily rather than social functioning, perhaps even to functional conditions of bodily parts. But it does not show that his definition should be rejected as such. Furthermore, even if Boorse's definition were shown by further counter-examples to be wholly invalid, this would not in itself invalidate the descriptivist approach to definition. For the invalidation of a particular descriptivist definition clearly does not in itself amount to an invalidation of descriptivism as a whole. Indeed, so far as medicine is concerned, the advantages of descriptivism (that I mentioned earlier) are such that the invalidation of Boorse's definition of 'dysfunction', far from undermining confidence in descriptivism, should act as a spur to the search for further and better descriptivist definitions.

NON-DESCRIPTIVIST: So you are saying that descriptivism is unfalsifiable!

Let me then return to the standard non-descriptivist objections to descriptivism. For these are not based on a mere accumulation of counter-examples to proposed descriptivist definitions of value terms. Such an accumulation, if not actually invalidating descriptivism, would at least make it less plausible. But non-descriptivist objections to descriptivism are based, rather, on the very logic of evaluation itself. According to non-descriptivism, the logical properties of value terms, as displayed in ordinary use, are such as to place difficulties of *principle* in the way of descriptivist definitions of them. If this is right, then it is no more possible to derive a value judgement solely from descriptive statements than it is to derive the number three, say, by adding just one plus one.

DESCRIPTIVIST: Give me an example, then. We had better start with a non-medical, and preferably a more or less

46

trivial example, in order to avoid confusing logical with substantive questions, questions of meaning with questions of fact or of value.

NON-DESCRIPTIVIST: Would you accept the value judgement 'This is a good strawberry'? We could then compare and contrast this with the description 'This is a wild strawberry'.

DESCRIPTIVIST: That's fine. And my first reaction is to point to a number of similarities between these two expressions which on the face of it seem to provide support for descriptivism.

In the first place, both expressions do convey descriptive meaning. In the second place, their descriptive meanings have several important logical properties in common. For example, the descriptive meanings of both are somewhat indeterminate: predicated of strawberries, 'good' could mean, severally or in combination, "plump", "sweet", "red" and so on; and 'wild' could mean, again severally or in combination, "small", "tasty", "fruiting all the year round" and so forth. Then again, the descriptive meanings of both expressions vary to some extent from one speaker to the next and from one occasion to the next. Also, both may be more or less vague. Hence, for all these and for other reasons, the descriptive meanings of both expressions may not be transparent.

NON-DESCRIPTIVIST: But closer inspection shows these similarities to be no more than superficial. The logical *significance* of the descriptive meanings conveyed by the two expressions is radically different. The descriptive meaning conveyed by 'wild' signifies the meaning of the *word* 'wild', whereas that conveyed by 'good' signifies something about people's taste in strawberries. That is to say, it signifies the criteria by which strawberries are judged to be good.

Thus, if in our example the descriptive meaning conveyed by 'wild' is taken to be "small and tasty", then 'wild' here means "small and tasty". But if the descriptive meaning conveyed by 'good' is taken to be "plump and sweet", then it is for the qualities of plumpness and sweetness that strawberries are being commended.

Similarly, if on other occasions other descriptive meanings are conveyed by 'wild', the word 'wild' is then being used with other meanings (for example, besides variations on 'wild' = "a particular species characterized, as above, by small, sweet fruit, produced all the year round", we find 'wild' = "uncultivated", "out of control" and so on). But if other descriptive meanings are conveyed by 'good' as used of strawberries, then it is for other qualities that strawberries are being commended. The *word* 'good', therefore, unlike the word 'wild', retains the same meaning (here, roughly, = "commendable") whatever descriptive meaning is conveyed by it. This is nicely shown by the limiting case in our example, that in which the descriptive meaning conveyed by 'good' is "wild"; for this would be a case of wild strawberries being commended, not a case of the word 'good' being used as a purely descriptive term synonymous with the word 'wild'.

The essential logical difference between the descriptive meanings conveyed by the two kinds of expression, descriptive and evaluative, comes out particularly clearly in disagreements. Thus disagreement about the descriptive meaning conveyed by 'wild' would be, straightforwardly, a disagreement about the meaning of the word 'wild'. It would be a disagreement about a logical issue, an issue of meaning. It would be a disagreement to be resolved by appealing to a dictionary, say. But a disagreement about the descriptive meaning conveyed by 'good' would be, or would ordinarily be taken to be, a disagreement about the qualities which make for good strawberries. Such a disagreement would thus not be a disagreement about the *meaning* of the word 'good' at all and could not usefully be referred to a dictionary. It would be a disagreement, rather, about a *substantive* (if trivial) question of value.

I have gone on a bit, but my point is that by observations such as these, we are led away from descriptivism to non-descriptivism, away from the view that value judgements are, or may be, derived logically (by entailment or such like) from descriptions, to the view that these two kinds of expression are entirely distinct logical species.

DESCRIPTIVIST: But they must be related somehow ...

NON-DESCRIPTIVIST: Certainly, but the *non*-descriptivist view is that, whatever their relationship, it is not possible to go from purely descriptive premises to evaluative conclusions.

This, I agree, is an essentially negative point. It says something about how description and evaluation are *not* related! Just how they are related is certainly a larger question. One idea is that the relationship is better understood perhaps as one of adoption rather than one of entailment. The descriptivist view is that value judgements may be entailed by descriptions. This particular non-descriptivist view, by contrast, is that descriptions are adopted as criteria *for* value judgements. According to this latter view, the description comes first, and then, as an entirely distinct and fully independent logical step, the adoption of the description as a criterion for a value judgement.

It is because of this extra step that, as I put it earlier, it is no more possible to derive a value judgement solely from descriptions than it is to derive the number three by adding one plus one.

DESCRIPTIVIST: That is, I suppose, more or less the line taken by the Oxford philosopher R. M. Hare in his books *The language of morals* (1952) and *Freedom and reason* (1963b), among other places.

But it has often been pointed out against Hare that if description and evaluation are really as independent as all that, then *any* criterion should do equally well for *any* value judgement, which is plainly not so. If the *only* link between a given criterion for a value judgement and the value judgement itself is that that criterion just *happens* to have been adopted for that value judgement, then any *other* criterion might just as well have been adopted instead.

That our choice of criteria should be in this way *wholly* unrestricted is perhaps just about plausible in some instances, particularly, as in your "good-strawberry" case, where the substantive issues are trivial. Certainly, it is true enough that people's taste in strawberries varies; and likewise that strawberries may themselves be valued other than as food. So there is much scope for variation in the criteria by which strawberries are evaluated – even a poisonous strawberry is a good strawberry for poisoning! All the same, for most value judgements, there will surely be at least some criteria the adoption of which would not make any sense at all.

This point has been made by another Oxford philosopher, G. J. Warnock in his book *Contemporary moral philosophy* (1967). Description and evaluation may well be logically independent, he writes, but this "does not imply, nor is it the case that, just anything can function as an (intelligible) criterion of evaluation" (p. 67). And, returning to medicine, this is surely the case where 'dysfunction' is used as a value term in clinical contexts. Take kidney-function, for example. It would not make any sense at all – it would not be intelligible – to adopt retention of waste products, say, rather than their excretion, as a criterion of good kidney-functioning.

NON-DESCRIPTIVIST: But Warnock, although he argues elsewhere as a descriptivist, is not in that particular reference denying the *logical* independence of description and evaluation. His point is rather that even if description and evaluation are independent in the way suggested by Hare, the interest and importance of this in moral (and other kinds of ethical) reasoning should not be exaggerated.

And Hare would not disagree with that. Certainly, it is no part of his view that just any criterion will do for any value judgement. Indeed, that this is *not* so is the nub of much of *Freedom and reason* and of his more recent book *Moral reasoning* (1981a). For, as Hare points out, regardless of whether there are *logical* constraints on the criteria which may be adopted for a particular value judgement, there are certainly *psychological* constraints. In my "good-strawberry" case, for example, no logical error would have been involved in judging a green, sour strawberry to be a good (dessert) strawberry. But greenness and sourness would have been "intelligible" as criteria of merit in (dessert) strawberries only to someone whose psychological make-up was such that he had a taste for green, sour strawberries. If anyone has such a taste, well and good. But, logical freedom or not, it is not possible in evaluating strawberries, or in making any other value judgement, simply to ignore our psychological make-up as given.

DESCRIPTIVIST: But surely the unintelligibility of retention of waste products as a criterion of good kidney-functioning, is not just a matter of psychology. Surely it is a matter of logic as well, a matter of the very meaning of 'good kidney-functioning'.

NON-DESCRIPTIVIST: I have to say, yes and no!

Yes, in the sense that it may well be right that retention of waste products is an intelligible criterion only of *bad* kidney-functioning, and that this is so for *logical*, rather than merely psychological, reasons. But also no, in the sense that there is no advantage in this for the descriptivist. For how is the term 'waste' to be defined without introducing a value judgement? And if 'waste' cannot be defined value-free, then the *non*-descriptivist principle remains intact. For the value judgement 'bad kidney-functioning' has then not been defined descriptively, but in terms of another value judgement, 'waste'.

This notion of a suppressed evaluative premiss, by the way, is directly relevant to some of the conceptual difficulties encountered in clinical medicine [see in particular chapter 6, in which the argument about 'kidney-functioning' is developed further, and chapter 7 on 'illness' and 'action'].

DESCRIPTIVIST: Well suppose we substitute for 'waste' a biological descriptive term such as 'urea'.

NON-DESCRIPTIVIST: But the effect of this would be merely to obscure still further the value judgement inherent in 'waste'. For, of course, not just any biological descriptive term will do. It will have to be one which describes a biochemical (or other material) which is judged to *be* waste. Indeed, this value judgement 'waste', is built into the very meaning of the term 'kidney'.

This is a difficult area [examined further in chapter 6], but the point, essentially, is this: 'kidney' *means* "organ with the function of excreting waste products"; therefore, in *calling* an organ a kidney, we are indeed committed by *logical* considerations, by the *meaning* of the word 'kidney', to certain limits on the criteria by which that organ can be judged to be functioning well or badly; hence, to judge a kidney which is retaining, rather than excreting, waste products, to be functioning well would indeed be, as you say, logically unintelligible, for it would be self-contradictory; but this fails to establish the descriptivist thesis, for the required logical considerations go back to the evaluative notion of 'waste' inherent in the definition of 'kidney'!

DESCRIPTIVIST: We seem to be falling back on very abstract, very theoretical considerations. But is there any practical point in all this for medicine?

If the criteria for those value judgements important in medicine are in practice determined by psychological and, to some extent, logical considerations, does it really matter, at the end of the day, whether description and evaluation are logically independent? In medicine, descriptivism may provide only an approximation to the (logical) truth, but it is a good approximation none the less – so good and so commonsensical in fact that the truths of non-descriptivism, if truths they be, are surely otiose.

NON-DESCRIPTIVIST: Not at all! It is the truths of descriptivism which in this context are otiose, and *because* they are commonsensical.

Look at it this way. In medicine, the truths of descriptivism are the common sense of medical *science*. But there is more to medicine than just science. And in this discussion, and in the wider debate, it is with the *non*-scientific aspects of medicine that we are largely concerned. Thus descriptivism is no more likely to be helpful here than is science itself [cf. chapter 2], while mere common sense of a vaguely "scientific" kind is likely to be positively misleading – all the more so if it is philosophically disguised.

DESCRIPTIVIST: Yet are there any indications that non-descriptivism will prove more useful in medicine than descriptivism?

NON-DESCRIPTIVIST: I believe that there are at least two indications, one general and one specific.

The general indication is this: that the overall attitude of the non-descriptivist to non-empirical problems in medicine is likely to be more direct, more square on, than that of the descriptivist.

Descriptivists will tend to ignore or side-step or diminish the importance of non-empirical problems in medicine. It is not necessary that they do so; but their central message, that value judgements may be analysed descriptively, is all too easily translated as a reductionist message in medical contexts – the message that non-empirical (as well as empirical) problems in medicine should be tackled, if at all, scientifically. Certainly some such message runs through most medical models. Boorse's arguments illustrate this rather well. His objective is to distil what he regards as a *properly* value-free concept of 'disease'; and his practical purpose thereby amounts to disentangling medicine *from*, rather than to resolving, the social and ethical issues listed at the beginning of his paper.

But the approach of the non-descriptivist to the same issues is likely to be more positive, less dismissive. The non-descriptivist is likely to take these issues seriously, as issues to be tackled *within* medicine, not as issues to be excluded from it. The non-descriptivist, furthermore, is likely to take these issues on their own terms, as *non*-empirical issues, and hence as issues which are no more to be dealt with as empirical issues (by a clearer or more determined application of science) than, in logic, values are to be dealt with as facts.

DESCRIPTIVIST: You mentioned that there was also a more specific indication of the potential usefulness of non-descriptivism in medicine.

NON-DESCRIPTIVIST: Yes, though this, too, has to do with the different approaches of descriptivism and non-descriptivism to questions of value.

53

The point, so far as medicine is concerned, is that non-descriptivism provides a far richer theoretical resource than descriptivism for dealing with the ethical problems of clinical practice.

The variation with context in the factual and evaluative connotations of value terms provides a good example of this. This variation is an important property of the medical value terms 'illness', 'disease', and 'dysfunction', being as it is at the heart of much of the present conceptual debate in medicine. Yet, as far as I am aware, only non-descriptivists such as Urmson (1950), and Hare (1952, Ch. 7) have paid much philosophical attention to it.

That this should be so is not surprising. For this property of value terms is one which is fully consistent with, and hence provides a degree of support for, non-descriptivism. And since it is a property of such importance in medicine, it is worth taking a brief look at why this should be so.

This is how the argument runs. According to non-descriptivists, the variation in the descriptive and evaluative connotations of value terms is a direct consequence of the way in which descriptive meaning becomes attached to value terms in the first place – that is, by adoption; the descriptive meaning conveyed by a value term being derived from the descriptive criteria adopted for the value judgement expressed by it. But it is a psychological fact that the criteria for some value judgements are more settled, more widely agreed upon, than the criteria for other value judgements. To revert to my earlier example, the criteria for 'good' use of strawberries, although variable, are none the less more settled, more widely agreed upon, than the criteria for 'good' use of paintings, say. It thus follows that the descriptive meanings conveyed by some value terms (or by some uses of the same value term) will be more prominent (because clearer and more self-evident) than the descriptive meanings conveyed by other value terms. Hence, for this and other similar reasons (discussed in the literature I referred to a moment ago) the strength of the descriptive connotations of value terms will vary with context.

Of course, this explanation leaves open the psychological

question of why the criteria for value judgements should vary in this way. But given the psychology, the logic (the non-descriptivist logic) follows. And it is this logic which has useful applications in medicine. (See chapters 4 and 5).

DESCRIPTIVIST: So we are to accept, against Boorse, that a value-free science of health is impossible. But medicine has advanced enormously through its development as a scientific discipline. What comfort, then, are you able to offer medicine?

NON-DESCRIPTIVIST: Only that no comfort is required.

Non-descriptivism is not prejudicial to science in medicine. On the contrary, by dispelling the misconception that medicine is nothing *more* than a science, non-descriptivism makes possible a more precise understanding of the proper role of science *within* medicine.

This is a large question, certainly [taken up in chapter 12]. But in reply to Boorse, it must now be clear that if all that is required is merely to preserve the status quo, the contortions of the "medical" model are wholly unnecessary. The foundation of a value-free science of health – at least of the kind which has proved so effective in physical medicine – is not a value-free definition of 'dysfunction', but, simply, value-free information regarding bodily functioning. Science itself may not be wholly value-free. But in so far as it is, there is no reason for it not to be value-free in medicine. And it is non-descriptivism, rather than descriptivism, which, by disentangling rather than compounding fact and value, is the more likely to make it so.

After all, it is well recognized in science that questions of value should not be confused with questions of fact. At its most elementary, then, the message of non-descriptivism is simply that the converse is also true: that in ethics, questions of fact (although nearly always relevant) should not be confused with questions of value. Keeping the two kinds of question distinct is thus just a first step towards dealing with either satisfactorily.

DESCRIPTIVIST: Though it must finally be admitted – to

finish on a point on which we can agree – that in dealing with questions of value, there is as yet no clear methodological counterpart to the scientific method which is available for dealing with questions of fact!

4
Disease

Implicit in the line of argument now developing are two shifts of emphasis away from those aspects of the conceptual structure of medicine conventionally regarded as important: a shift, mainly in chapter 2, from 'disease' – and the relationship between it and 'dysfunction' – to 'illness'; and a shift, mainly in chapter 3, from the factual to the evaluative connotations of these terms. In this chapter, these two shifts of emphasis will be brought together. The relationship between 'disease' and 'illness' will be interpreted in terms of the evaluative logical element in their meanings. This interpretation will turn out quite differently from any conventional interpretation. In the literature generally, as in Boorse's theory, because 'disease' is prominent and important in medicine, 'illness', with its more marked evaluative connotations, has been interpreted as a derivative concept. Here, on the contrary, it will be found that 'disease' is the derivative concept and that its properties, including its prominence and importance as a mainly factual term in medicine, are to a large extent actually determined by the properties of 'illness' as a value term.

The strategy to be followed is this: first, the idea that 'illness' is a value term will be adopted as an assumption; next, a hypothesis about 'disease' will be derived from this assumption; finally, this hypothesis will be developed to give an interpretation of the relationship between 'disease' and 'illness'. This interpretive stage will occupy most of the chapter. But its success will substantiate the hypothesis about 'disease' and, in turn, the original assumption about 'illness'.

Assumption about illness

The initial assumption, then, is that 'illness' is a value term; or, more exactly, that the central use of 'illness', as a term distinct in meaning from 'disease', is to express a (negative) value judgement. It follows, therefore, from what was said in chapter 3, that with this use of 'illness' will go criteria for the value judgement that is expressed by it. But the criteria for value judgements, as we saw, vary with context, for some value judgements more and for others less widely, from time to time, from person to person and from place to place. The assumption that 'illness' is a value term is thus fully consistent with the fact of ordinary usage noted in chapter 2, that the criteria for 'illness' vary in just this way. It is true that the criteria for 'illness', unlike those for general-purpose value terms such as 'good' and 'bad', are not wholly unrestricted. That is to say, *any* condition *may* be negatively evaluated; and, if our assumption about 'illness' is right, a condition can be an illness only if it is a negatively evaluated condition; but not *every* negatively evaluated condition is an illness; to be an illness a negatively evaluated condition must be, *inter alia*, a condition of a living as opposed to a non-living thing and a condition typically, though not necessarily exclusively, of persons. Still, granted all this, it remains true that among those conditions that *may* be construed as illnesses, there are some that are more and others that are less widely construed in this way. And this variation is both consistent with the assumption that 'illness' is a value term, and, if this assumption is correct, at least partly explained by it.

A full specification of the requirements for a condition to be an illness would amount to an analysis of 'illness'. The development of such a specification will occupy much of parts III and IV. In these later parts our approach will be to consider the particular kind of negative value that is expressed by 'illness' and how an examination of this may help to explain the origins of some of the non-empirical clinical problems with which this book is concerned. In the present chapter, however, it is the variation as such, in how widely or consistently different conditions are regarded as illnesses, that is important.

For it is from this variation that our hypothesis about 'disease' will be derived; and it is from the identification of this variation (under our initial assumption) as a variation in the criteria for the value judgement expressed by 'illness', that an interpretation of the relationship between 'illness' and 'disease' will be developed.

Hypothesis about disease

If some conditions are more and others less widely construed as illnesses, two categories of conditions may be defined: a category, I, of conditions that *may* be construed as illnesses, and a subcategory of I consisting of conditions that are *widely* construed as such. It is from the *sub*category that the present hypothesis about 'disease' will (shortly) be derived. The subcategory will therefore be called Id. Membership of I is determined by the requirements for a condition to be an illness, requirements which have so far been defined only in part. Membership of Id depends on how wide is 'widely'. Any exact definition of Id will to some extent be arbitrary, since the variation in how widely different conditions are construed as illnesses is really continuous, rather than categorical. But an exact definition is not required here anyway. For our hypothesis about 'disease' is simply that, in so far as it is a term distinct in meaning from 'illness', it is to the members of Id that it refers. And indeed, if the boundary of Id (defined by 'widely') is an inexact boundary, this is fully consistent with the inexact boundary between 'illness' and 'disease' in ordinary usage (again, as noted in chapter 2).

Our hypothesis is also inexact in a second respect. It claims that 'disease' *refers* to the members of Id. But in what sense "refers"? Drawing on the key distinction considered in chapter 3, to refer could be to state facts and/or to express value judgements. But it could also be to make claims (for example scientific or political claims), to explain, to issue instructions, to vilify and so on. Engelhardt (1986), Merskey (1986) and others have emphasized the variety of purposes that medical language may serve. And in interpreting 'disease', it is clearly as important to understand the *kind* of reference made by it as to know that to which it refers.

The inexactness of 'refers', however, like that of 'widely', is appropriate here. For 'disease' itself is inexact. Just as the term 'refer' is non-specific, there being many different kinds of reference, so also is 'disease'. As we saw in chapter 2, there are many different kinds of disease, many varieties of disease category, as well as historical and diagnostic shifts between them. In some contexts, 'disease' is close in meaning to 'illness'; in others it is contrasted with it. Mostly it has factual connotations, but it may also have evaluative connotations. The use, therefore, of the non-specific term 'refers' in our hypothesis about 'disease' at least makes it possible that this hypothesis can encompass all these varieties and variations. And more precise definition of the way or ways in which 'disease' refers to the members of Id will thus amount also to more precise definition of 'disease'.

Development of the hypothesis to explain the relationship between disease and illness

Our hypothesis about 'disease' will now be developed by looking at some of the possible ways in which 'disease' could refer to the members of Id. In ordinary usage, however, as noted in chapter 2, the varieties and variations of 'disease' are not clearly distinguished, but are often combined and overlapping. Rather than attempting to draw directly on ordinary usage, therefore, we will come to it indirectly. That is to say, rather than attempting to analyse ordinary usage we will consider a series of *prima-facie* likely ways in which 'disease' *might* "refer" to the members of Id. For each of these hypothetical uses of 'disease' (or HDs), we will ask how, given the relationship between Id and I, the relationship between that particular HD and 'illness' would appear in or as part of ordinary usage. And the combined appearances of these hypothetical relationships, severally and together, should therefore, if our hypothesis about 'disease' is correct, correspond to the appearance in ordinary usage of the relationship between 'disease' and 'illness'.

HDv: hypothetical use of 'disease' as a value term

Possibly the most straightforward way in which 'disease' might refer to conditions in Id would be by expressing the value judgement in relation to which these conditions, by definition, stand as criteria. But this is also the value judgement which is expressed by 'illness'. In this case, then, not only would 'disease' express a value judgement, it would express the same value judgement as 'illness'. According to our hypothesis, however, 'disease' would be used only of conditions in Id, while 'illness' could be used of conditions in I as a whole. The relationship between HDv and 'illness' would thus be similar to the relationship between 'disease' and 'illness' in ordinary usage, as described in chapter 2, to the extent that, although (1) HDv could sometimes be used as a synonym for 'illness', that is, of conditions in Id; and although (2) the two terms would always be closely linked, being used in similar contexts, with similar implications, and so on; none the less, (3) there would be circumstances in which they could not be used as synonyms, i.e., of conditions in I that are not in Id; though, since the boundary of Id is not well defined, (4) synonymous and non-synonymous uses would not always be clearly distinct.

The restriction of HDv to conditions in Id would result also in a fifth, perhaps more important similarity between it and the ordinary use of 'disease'. For this restriction would result in HDv, like 'disease' in ordinary usage, having less overtly evaluative connotations (a less clearly evaluative "ring" to it) than 'illness'. This follows from an important property of value terms noted in chapter 3: namely, that the strength of the evaluative connotations of a value term varies inversely with the extent to which the criteria for the value judgement expressed by it are settled or agreed – the *more* settled the criteria, the *less* marked (by and large) are its evaluative connotations. But to say (as in chapter 3) that the criteria for a value judgement are widely settled or agreed, is just another way of saying (as in this chapter) that conditions in Id are widely construed as illnesses. Hence, although HDv and 'illness' are both value terms, and although both express the same value judgement, the restriction of HDv to conditions in Id will result in its evaluative connotations being less marked than those of 'illness'. Indeed, to draw the same conclusion rather more strongly, it is by *virtue* of the properties that HDv and 'illness' have in common *as* value terms, that HDv would have less, and 'illness' more, marked evaluative connotations.

Five similarities have thus been identified between HDv and 'disease' in ordinary usage. It is not unlikely, therefore, that uses of 'disease' along the lines of HDv might contribute to ordinary usage. And certainly, among the varieties and admixtures of ordinary usage, examples of 'disease' looking very like HDv are readily distinguishable. This, consistently with the present hypothesis is most clearly so where 'illness' and 'disease' are used as synonyms or near synonyms. An example of this was given in chapter 2. It was noted that the expression "some awful illness" could in many contexts be rendered without change of meaning as "some awful disease". Moreover, consistently with HDv, 'disease' in contexts of this kind has clear evaluative force. But 'disease' is only fully interchangeable with 'illness', as HDv would only be fully interchangeable with 'illness', in respect of conditions widely regarded as illnesses. If someone has a hangover, for example, then, as noted in chapter 2, while they might be said to be ill, they would not normally be said to have a disease. And the reason for this, if our hypothesis about 'disease' is correct, is that while the condition of being hung-over is a bad condition to be in, there is some uncertainty (for reasons which will become apparent in chapters 7 and 8) as to whether it is a bad condition of the kind properly construed as an illness. Hangovers, that is to say, are at best on the edge of Id.

HDf: hypothetical use of 'disease' as a factual term

A number of different hypothetical uses of 'disease' as a factual term are possible. The simplest of these will be considered first, HDf1. The simplest way in which 'disease', used as a factual term might "refer" to conditions in Id would be just to *describe* them as diseases – namely, as conditions widely held as criteria for the value judgement expressed by 'illness'; or, less long-windedly, as conditions widely construed as illnesses.

HDf1, then, would state a *fact* rather than express an evaluation; it would describe *how* a condition is evaluated (that is, negatively, as an illness), rather than evaluating it as such. Thus, following chapter 3, HDf1 would be a term of an entirely different logical kind from both 'illness' and HDv. Unlike HDv, HDf1 could never properly be used as a synonym for 'illness', and it would be in this respect unlike the employments of 'disease' *as* HDv in ordinary usage. HDf1, however, would be similar to HDv in each of the four other respects in which HDv is similar to 'disease' in ordinary usage, though in part for different reasons. Thus (first similarity), HDf1 would be closely linked with 'illness'; by context, in that both terms are used of conditions in Id, and by (certain) implications, in that a reference to 'illness' is entailed by the use of HDf1. However (second similarity), since HDf1 and 'illness' are terms of different logical kinds, they would necessarily be distinct in meaning. Though (third similarity), since facts about evaluations and expressions of value are not always clearly distinguished, HDf1 and 'illness' would not always be clearly distinguished. Nonetheless (fourth similarity), since HDf1 essentially states a fact, whereas 'illness' expresses a value judgement, HDf1 would have less, and 'illness' more, marked evaluative connotations.

In addition to these shared similarities, HDf1, being a factual term, would show certain further similarities to 'disease' in ordinary usage. These further similarities, indeed, are best understood by reference to the differences between factual terms and value terms generally in the purposes for which they are respectively employed in ordinary usage. Thus, as emphasized in 'emotivist' ethical theory (for example, Ayer, 1936; Stevenson, 1945), a statement of fact is typically used to change what is known, whereas expressions of value are typically used to evince or evoke feelings and/or emotions, to change attitudes and to provoke action. Thus, HDf1, being a factual term, would be similar to 'disease' in ordinary usage in that, as described in chapter 2, it would be used typically, as by doctors making diagnoses, to say *what* is wrong with someone who is ill. And it would in this respect differ, as 'disease' in ordinary usage differs, from the evaluative term 'illness', which is used typically, as by patients or their relatives, to evince or evoke concern, to change unsympathetic attitudes and to provoke therapeutic action. HDfi, like 'disease', would thus be broadly for doctors, whereas 'illness' is broadly for patients and their relatives; the former having the more technical, the latter the more personal connotations. Similarly, HDfi, like 'disease', and unlike 'illness', would be used equally of animals and plants as of people, since it is mainly for people that we feel concern merely *that* something is wrong, whereas for all three equally – for animals and plants as well as for people – we may be concerned with *what*, factually speaking, *is* wrong. And the rule-proving exception here, domestic animals and plants, fits nicely, in that our concerns for these are often similar to the concerns that we have for people.

Given, then, so many similarities between HDfi and 'disease' in ordinary usage, it is no surprise to find, besides HDv-like uses of 'disease', HDfi-like uses as well. Examples of the latter are most obvious, perhaps, in respect of those conditions described in chapter 2 as 'symptomatically' defined diseases. Migraine was the example given there. If someone has migraine, they may be said to be ill. And, consistently with our initial assumption about 'illness', this is most likely to be said in non-technical contexts with evaluative force – for example, as an expression of concern. But in more technical contexts, as in making a diagnosis, someone with migraine would be said simply, and as a matter of fact, to *have* migraine. And by this would be implied both that they have a particular condition (a characteristic headache, and so on) and that they have a condition which is widely construed as an illness. Normally the latter implication can be taken for granted in practice. But both implications are in principle necessary if 'migraine' is to serve as an adequate (medical) answer to the diagnostic question, what is wrong: the former (that they have a particular condition) because it tells us what *can* be done about the patient's condition, the latter (that that condition is widely construed as an illness) because it tells us that what can be done would be widely regarded as what *ought* (medically) to be done. Both implications are thus necessary to decisions about treatment;

and it is with the latter that HDf1-like uses of the concept of 'disease' are identifiable.

Decisions about treatment, however, as described in chapter 2, although served to some extent by symptomatically defined diseases, are served rather better by diseases which are causally defined. And it will now be clear, having identified HDf1 with the former, that a second hypothetical use of 'disease' as a factual term can be identified with the latter – namely, a use of 'disease' which describes a condition not as one which *is* widely regarded as an illness (HDf1), but as one which is a *cause* of a condition which is widely regarded as an illness (HDf2). HDf2, being – like HDf1 – a factual term, would show all the same similarities to 'disease' in ordinary usage. But it would show one further similarity as well. This arises from the fact (discussed for example by Ayer, 1976, Ch. vii) that causal connections, such as those implied by HDf2, between conditions denoted by this use of 'disease' and conditions in the subcategory Id, need to be no more than connections of tendency: that is to say, for A to be considered a cause of B, it is not necessary that B should always follow *immediately* upon A, nor even that B should *always* follow upon A at all, but only that B should *tend* to folow A (though this is not a sufficient condition for A to be a cause of B). It thus follows that if one's condition is such that, although not actually ill, one is likely to become ill, then in the HDf2-sense of the term, one may be said to have a disease even though one is not ill. HDf2 (and other similar secondary senses of 'disease') can thus have a degree of independence in ordinary usage from their logical parent, 'illness'. Although derived from 'illness', 'disease' in its HDf2 sense has a life of its own. And this of course corresponds with cases in ordinary usage in which one is said to have a disease even though one is not ill, asymptomatic cases of diabetes and cancer, for example, as described in chapter 2.

It is in terms of HDf2, also, that many of the features of 'dysfunction' in ordinary (medical) usage and of its relationship with 'disease' (though not with 'illness') may be understood. For if a functional condition, of the body at least, is a cause of a condition which is widely regarded as an illness, then, in the HDf2-sense of the term, it *is* a disease. But, as we saw in chapter 2, not all functional conditions, not even all functional conditions of the body, not even all negatively evaluated functional conditions of the body, are causes of illness. Likewise, not all causes of illness are negatively evaluated functional bodily conditions. In these respects, then, HDf2-diseases, in so far as they are defined in terms of dysfunctional bodily conditions, would be consistent with the corresponding features of 'disease' in ordinary usage. Thus, although some HDf2-diseases would be defined in terms of negatively evaluated functional conditions of the body, not all such dysfunctional conditions would be diseases, neither would all diseases be so defined. Furthermore, if the relationship between 'dysfunction' and 'disease' is understood this way, Flew's constraint, as described in chapter 2, is satisfied. For the class of dysfunctional bodily conditions in terms of which (HDf2-like) diseases may be defined is definitely circumscribed – that is to say, by the value judgement expressed by 'illness'. Finally, if the relationship between 'dysfunction' and 'disease' is understood this way, the bridge of meaning between 'dysfunction' and 'illness' formed by 'disease' in ordinary usage is explained, straightforwardly, by the series HDf2 ... HDf1 ... HDv.

Turning to the (direct) relationship between 'dysfunction' and 'illness', on the other hand, the logical non-equivalence of these two concepts noted in chapter 2 remains something of a mystery. It is true, of course, that in so far as causes generally are distinct from their effects, illness-causing dysfunctional conditions (as a subgroup of HDf2-diseases) are distinct from the illnesses which are their effects. But not all dysfunctional bodily conditions and illnesses are distinct in this way. Finding, for example, that one's legs suddenly fail to function properly – that they just give way, say, or that they move when they should not move – one could well take oneself to be ill. That is to say, the *same* condition is here capable of being construed either as a dysfunctional condition or an illness. Yet the two construals are not strictly equivalent. For it is one's *legs* which are not functioning properly, but one's *self* who is ill. This, then, is a feature of ordinary usage which has not been explained by our analysis so far. Still, it is one which is also not explained by other available analyses. In particular, it is not explained by the "medical" model (chapter 2). Furthermore, as will be seen in chapter 7, it is at least partly explained by the present analysis once the latter has been extended to encompass more fully the meanings of 'dysfunction' and 'illness'.

HDf2 also helps us in one further respect, however, by suggesting further hypothetical uses of 'disease'. Thus the reference to conditions in the subcategory Id implied by HDf2, is an indirect rather than a direct reference, since conditions denoted by HDf1 are conditions *in* Id, whereas conditions denoted by HDf2 are merely *causes* of conditions in Id. But an indirect reference to conditions in Id is made possible not only by the causal relationship implied by HDf2 but by any relationship whatsoever. By analogy with HDf2, therefore, many further hypothetical uses of 'disease' are possible, at least in principle. In practice, of course, only those which are useful will actually be employed. But even in medicine, let alone other contexts (for example, medico-legal contexts), these are various enough. Many diseases, for example, particularly in physical medicine, are defined, at least in part and at least in the first instance, by clinical signs and/or laboratory test results, the relationships of which to the symptoms of illness are statistical rather than causal – for example, secondary syphilis is defined in part by characteristic, but in themselves often symptomless (as, say, sun-induced freckles are symptomless) skin rashes. However, since knowledge of the causes of illness is, on the whole, more useful in medicine than other kinds of knowledge, for this reason alone and not for any reason of conceptual priority, the causal sense of 'disease' will come to predominate over other senses as and when such knowledge becomes available.

Implications

The view of 'disease' and 'illness' and of the relationship between them which has now been set out is in important respects the reverse of the conventional view. This reverse view, however, has turned out to be both more complicated (in its analysis of 'disease') and less familiar than the conventional view. Is it then justified?

It is justified, first, under the first outcome criterion described at the end of chapter 1, in that it explains the features of the ordinary usage of 'illness', 'disease' and 'dysfunction' more comprehensively than any conventional view. The features of the ordinary usage of the medical terms which are explained by the conventional view are mainly those which are prominent in technical contexts in medicine. Indeed, these features, as we saw in chapter 2, are the very basis of the conventional view. In technical contexts, 'disease', used with mainly factual connotations and defined as far as possible in terms of 'dysfunction', is far more prominent than the evaluative 'illness'. Hence, according to the conventional view, the conceptual root notion in medicine must be 'dysfunction', a (supposedly) value-free, biological-scientific concept from which 'disease' and, in turn, 'illness' are both derived. In non-technical contexts, the conventional view continues, it may well be that 'illness', and sometimes 'disease' used with evaluative connotations, are the more prominent concepts. Similarly, in such contexts, it may well be that, contrary to the (conventional) derivation of 'disease' from 'illness', one may be said to be ill without being said to have a disease. Furthermore, it may be that there are aspects of ordinary usage even in technical contexts (the relationship between 'dysfunction' and 'disease', for example), with which the conventional view is inconsistent. But all such usage is to be written off as merely primitive, as "two thousand years out of date", in the words of Boorse's 1976 paper (p. 76), since it ignores the development of medicine as a modern scientific discipline.

All, then, very different from our reverse view, which, as we have seen, accommodates the features of ordinary usage in non-technical contexts just as fully as its features in technical contexts. This is at the expense of a degree of complication, certainly; but then ordinary usage itself is complicated. According to our reverse view, 'illness', not 'dysfunction', is the conceptual root notion in medicine, conditions being first marked out as illnesses by the value judgement expressed by 'illness'. This value judgement has still to be analysed (in chapters 7 et seq.). But even without further analysis, a variety of hypothetical uses of 'disease' can be derived from it: an evaluative use (HDv) expressing the same value judgement as 'illness' but limited to conditions (in the subcategory Id) widely regarded as illness; and a series of factual uses, HDf1, HDf2 and HDf3. As it is, even these hypothetical uses by no means exhaust the possibilities. As already noted, there could be many other uses of 'disease' as a factual term. There could also be other uses of 'disease' as a value term; for example, in addition to HDv, 'disease' can be used non-specifically, implying simply a bad or unwelcome condition – though here the non-specific term 'sick' is more likely to be used. And there could be other uses of 'disease' altogether; for example, a persuasive use, persuading us that some condition *should* be regarded as an illness, as in the title of Jellinek's 1960 book arguing the case for alcoholism, *The disease concept of alcoholism*. However, it is uses of 'disease' corresponding with HDf1 (symptomatic), HDf2 (causal) and HDf3 (statistical) that are most prominent in technical contexts. And this, within a reverse view analysis, is for empirical reasons, not conceptual. It is for reasons to do with the usefulness of these concepts in relation to the empirical clinical problems with which doctors have been mainly concerned. Weight, therefore, the hypothetical uses of 'disease' described here with these empirical considerations; run them together with 'illness', allowing different shades of meaning, different combinations and permutations in different contexts; allow these different shades of meaning to be often less than fully explicit or even fully conscious; and the amalgam which is then produced corresponds very largely with ordinary usage.

Under our first outcome criterion, therefore, a reverse view is not so much justified despite the complications inherent in it, as actually endorsed by them. As to the unfamiliarity of this view, somewhat similar considerations apply under the second outcome criterion, the criterion of practical utility. In the first place, it will be recalled from chapter 2 that the conventional view is suspect as a basis for analytical research precisely because it is a familiar view. It is familiar because it is concerned with aspects of the conceptual structure of medicine prominent in technical contexts. But these aspects are prominent because of their utility in relation to *empirical* clinical problems, whereas analytical research in medicine is concerned primarily with *non*-empirical problems. Hence, in switching attention from the (conventionally) familiar to other aspects of the conceptual structure of medicine, a reverse view is at least not suspect in this particular regard.

However, a more important point to make in respect of the practical utility of a reverse view is that outside technical contexts, it, or its conceptual elements at least, are really not unfamiliar at all. Indeed, although the conventional view has been described here as based on aspects of the conceptual structure of medicine prominent in technical contexts in medicine, it would be more accurate to describe it as based on those aspects of the conceptual structure of medicine prominent in technical contexts just in hospital-based physical medicine. It is here that scientific progress in medicine has been most dramatic in recent years. And it has been in connection with this progress that mainly factual uses of 'disease' and 'dysfunction' have been prominent – hence the tendency to suppose that these uses of these concepts are somehow, as in the conventional view, also *logically* basic. But outside of hospital-based physical medicine, 'illness', and value-laden uses of the medical concepts generally, are not unfamiliar at all. This is true, notably, as emphasized already in this chapter, of patients. And for patients, at least, the logical priority of 'illness' (a key feature of any reverse view) corresponds with the actual *experience* of illness; for the complaint normally precedes the diagnosis of the complaint; knowledge *that* something is wrong normally precedes the question *what* is wrong, let alone questions about possible *causes* of what is wrong.

There will be more to say about all this in chapter 11, in which the elements of a reverse view, shown here on theoretical grounds to be logically primary, will be found also to be the elements familiar in that whole area of practical medicine called "primary" health care. But, more immediately, it is important to recognize that these are also the elements familiar in psychological medicine. In psychological medicine it is 'mental *illness*', not 'mental disease', that is the more familiar concept. In psychological medicine, too, it is with 'mental *illness*' that the non-empirical problems with which analytical research is concerned are associated. The debate in the literature, after all, is a debate about 'mental *illness*'. And much of this debate has been concerned with the evaluative connotations of this term. Of course, none of this amounts to "proof" that a reverse view is right and the conventional view wrong. On the contrary, we will find in chapter 12 that a reverse view, once it has been fully worked out, is better understood as placing the conventional view in a broader and more complete conceptual context. Nevertheless, it is encouraging at this stage of the argument to find that in addition to its better correspondence with ordinary usage, a reverse view emphasizes those elements of the conceptual structure of medicine most closely associated with the non-empirical problems of clinical practice.

5

Illness

Notwithstanding its *prima-facie* relevance to psychological medicine, the reverse view of the medical concepts set out in chapter 4 was developed mainly with physical medicine in mind. This is consistent with the general approach settled in chapter 1, namely that the analysis, although concerned ultimately with problems raised largely by 'mental illness', should proceed in the first instance from examples of physical illness. In fact, relatively little was said about 'illness', either physical or mental, in chapter 4. Most of that chapter, corresponding with ordinary usage in physical medicine, was taken up with 'disease'. The place of 'illness' was pivotal, it is true; since it was from 'illness', as a kind of conceptual germ-cell, that the various disease concepts, HDv, HDf1, HDf2 and so on, were derived. But all that was required of 'illness' for these derivations was that it be a (negative) value term.

This *de minimis* interpretation of 'illness', however, is not likely to be sufficient when the analysis moves on from physical medicine to psychological. Indeed, it will be recalled from chapter 1 that there are two requirements in particular that a reverse view (or any other analysis of the medical concepts) must satisfy in advance of just this move: first, that it should show whether there is a general concept, 'illness', distinct from 'physical illness'; second, that in so doing it should explain, or be capable of explaining, both the similarities and the differences between 'physical illness' and 'mental illness'. What is needed now, therefore, is a progress report, an assessment of the extent to which the reverse view developed in chapter 4 meets these two requirements. This is the task of the present chapter. From it will come a clearer picture of what must be added to the analysis of 'illness' before we can move on to 'mental illness'.

Requirement 1

In respect of our first requirement – that the analysis show whether there is a general concept of 'illness' – the reverse view developed in chapter 4, although as yet providing no firm conclusion, suggests a number of relevant points. Thus, in chapter 1 the term 'illness' was used generically, to include 'disease' and (the medical uses of) 'dysfunction'. It is now clear, however, in the more specific terminology of chapter 4, that if 'illness' is the prior concept in medicine, as it is in any reverse view, then any move by generalization from physical medicine to psychological medicine is likely to be by way of 'illness' rather than 'disease' or 'dysfunction'. Then again, and similarly, it is also clear that the demonstration of a general concept, 'illness', distinct from 'physical illness', will come, if at all, from an analysis of 'physical illness' in its own right rather than, as so often in the literature, as a (supposed) derivative of 'disease' or 'dysfunction'. The comments on 'illness' made at the start of chapter 4 represent the beginnings of just such an analysis. And if this analysis has not as yet been taken very far, there are nevertheless two reasons for believing that it has at least been heading in the right general direction.

The first reason is that this analysis, although an analysis primarily of 'physical illness', is in principle fully generalizable to 'mental illness'. This is because the (minimal) specification noted in chapter 4 for a condition to be an illness is satisfied by at least some mental conditions: mental conditions may be, and centrally are, of living things; they are typically of persons; and they may be evaluated negatively (or, of course, positively). Furthermore, those mental conditions ordinarily thought of as mental illnesses actually *do* satisfy this specification. That is to say, mental illnesses, like physical illnesses, are (typically) negatively evaluated conditions of living persons. In itself this does not establish the validity of the concept of 'mental illness'. The specification of 'physical illness' given in chapter 4 is too broad to do that; after all, there are many other kinds of

negatively evaluated conditions of living persons besides illnesses. But at least everything said in chapter 4 about conditions
ordinarily thought of as physical illnesses can also be said about
conditions ordinarily thought of as mental illnesses. And at
least, therefore, there is nothing in chapter 4 which could act as
a barrier to the more specific generalization that will eventually
be required.

The second reason for believing that the analysis of chapter 4
is heading in the right general direction stems from the parallel
which exists between physical illnesses and mental illnesses in
the phenomena by which they are typically constituted. In
chapter 2 it was noted that whereas physical *diseases* are
constituted typically – though not exclusively – by changes in
bodily structure and function, physical *illnesses* are constituted
typically – though not exclusively – by feelings and sensations
such as pain. However, whereas changes in bodily structure and
function would ordinarily be thought of as physical phenomena, feelings and sensations would ordinarily be thought of as
mental phenomena. Hence, physical illnesses are constituted
typically by phenomena ordinarily thought of as mental
phenomena.

Now it would be wrong to make too much of this
observation. In the first place it raises a number of difficult
questions in general philosophy; questions about the relationship between mind and body, about the ordinary distinction
between 'mental' and 'physical' and so on. Secondly, as set out,
it begs the very question with which this book as a whole is
centrally concerned, namely what it is that illness (physical or
mental) actually consists in – just as not all changes in bodily
structure and function are constituents of disease (chapter 2), so
not all feelings and sensations are constituents of illness; and our
task here is to define the way or ways in which feelings and
sensations (along with other illness constituents) are marked out
as constituents of illness. Thirdly, even as stated, the observation does not in itself supply the general concept 'illness'
which we require. Nor does it establish the validity of 'mental
illness'; for mental illnesses are (in the sense of the term used
here) constituted typically by varieties of mental phenomena
quite different from those by which physical illnesses are

constituted: the mental illness constituents corresponding with feelings and sensations would include, for example, emotions, appetites, impulses and beliefs.

But granted all these reservations, what the observation does achieve, taken together with a reverse view of the medical concepts, is an uncoupling or detachment of the analysis of 'physical illness' from purely physical phenomena. As long as 'illness' is regarded as a derivative of 'disease', and as long as 'disease' is analysed in terms of the physical phenomena (the changes in bodily structure and function) by which it is typically constituted, then 'physical illness' will also be analysed in terms of physical phenomena – at one remove perhaps, but at the end of the day in terms of physical phenomena all the same. However, if 'illness' is the prior concept, and therefore to be analysed in its own right, an analysis of 'physical illness' is *de facto* an analysis of illness constituted by mental as well as physical phenomena. To this very limited extent, then, the present analysis has already moved closer to an analysis of 'mental illness'.

To sum up. In relation to the first requirement in chapter 1, there is nothing in the analysis so far to prevent there being a general concept, 'illness', distinct from 'physical illness'. Such a concept has not yet been demonstrated. But in recognizing the conceptual priority of 'illness' it has been shown that if a general concept exists, then it is likely to be found by further analysis of 'illness', rather than of 'disease' or 'dysfunction'. And with this in mind, the reverse-view analysis in chapter 4 is heading in the right direction, since it is both capable of, and has progressed some way towards, generalization from 'physical illness' to 'mental illness'.

Requirement 2

The second requirement set out in chapter 1 was that the analysis should explain, rather than explain away (as in the literature), both the similarities and the differences between the concepts employed in physical medicine and psychological medicine.

Similarities

One important conceptual difference between physical medicine and psychological medicine, to which attention was drawn at the end of chapter 4, is that whereas 'disease' is the more prominent concept in the former, 'illness' is the more prominent in the latter. In the literature, this difference has often been overlooked, essentially because the distinction between 'illness' and 'disease' has often been overlooked. This has led, somewhat paradoxically, to an exaggerated idea of the conceptual differences between physical and psychological medicine. For in failing to distinguish between 'illness' and 'disease', the tendency has been unwittingly to compare 'mental illness', the more prominent concept in psychological medicine, not with its proper counterpart in physical medicine, namely 'physical *illness*', but with 'physical *disease*'. Hence the properties of 'illness' have been attributed to what has been in effect the conflation 'mental illness/disease', while the properties of 'disease' have been attributed to the corresponding 'physical illness/disease'. 'Mental illness/disease', therefore, recalling the differences between 'illness' and 'disease' noted in chapter 2, has been regarded as relatively subjective and evaluative, whereas 'physical illness/disease' has been seen as relatively objective and factual.

Once 'illness' and 'disease' are clearly distinguished, however, it becomes possible to compare like with like, 'mental illness' with 'physical illness', 'mental disease' with 'physical disease'. And the conceptual differences between psychological and physical medicine are then seen to be much smaller than is commonly supposed. In the first place, as noted a moment ago, mental illnesses are like physical illnesses in satisfying the (necessary but not sufficient) specification outlined in chapter 4 for a condition to be an illness. Then again, and rather more significantly, physical illnesses are like mental illnesses in being constituted typically by mental, rather than physical, phenomena. But what can now be added to these similarities is that just as 'mental illness' is variable, subjective and value-laden, so too is 'physical illness'. The two kinds of illness differ quantitatively in these respects, it is true; 'mental illness' being more variable, subjective and value-laden than 'physical illness'. This, as will be seen in a moment, is one important consequence of their being constituted typically by different kinds of mental phenomena. But all the same, the differences are only quantitative, not qualitative.

Similar comments can be made about the differences between 'physical disease' and 'mental disease'. The concept of 'disease', though less prominent in psychological than physical medicine, is in both disciplines less subjective and value-laden than the concept of 'illness'. Similarly, mental-disease categories, for reasons we will come to shortly, are less well developed than physical-disease categories. But the three principal categories – defined respectively in terms of symptoms, associated conditions and causes (cf. chapter 4) – are the same in psychological as in physical medicine, albeit in different proportions.

Merely to distinguish 'illness' from 'disease' is thus to reduce the apparent conceptual gap between physical medicine and psychological medicine. What is made of this, however, will depend on what is made of the differences between 'illness' and 'disease' themselves. And it is here that a reverse view becomes important. In the literature, as noted in chapter 2, where 'illness' is distinguished from 'disease' at all, it is normally regarded as the less satisfactory concept, at least for technical or specialist use in medicine, precisely because it is the more subjective and value-laden. On this view, then, recognition of the fact that 'mental illness' is in these respects like 'physical illness' simply reinforces the idea prevalent in the literature, that the conceptual structure of psychological medicine is unsatisfactory in one way or another as compared with that of physical medicine. For, however close the concept of 'mental disease' is to that of 'physical disease', it is still 'mental *illness*', the (supposedly) *less* satisfactory concept, that is the *more* widely deployed in psychological medicine. And from this, it will be concluded, come the vagueness, the subjectivity and the value-laden nature of the subject. Analytical effort will therefore be directed, as in the debate about mental illness, towards what is perceived as putting matters to rights: either, as among the pro-psychiatry lobby, by emphasizing the conceptual similarities between physical medicine and psychological medicine at the expense of the differences; or, as among the anti-psychiatry lobby, by seeking to minimize these similarities to the point where psychological medicine can no longer be regarded as medicine at all.

According to a reverse view, however, neither 'illness' nor 'disease' is regarded as more or less "satisfactory". The priority afforded to 'illness' is a conceptual priority only. 'Illness' is prior to 'disease' only in the sense that the meaning of 'disease' is derived from that of 'illness', not vice versa. On this view, therefore, there is no reason either to exaggerate or minimize the conceptual similarities between physical and psychological medicine. These similarities have still to be explained (in terms of our yet to be demonstrated general concept). But in advance of explanation, a reverse view, unlike any conventional view, is at least a neutral view.

Differences

Much the same can be said of the differences between the two kinds of medicine. Just as a reverse view is neutral with regard to the similarities, so it is neutral with regard to the differences between them. Both are phenomena to be explained, rather than explained away. This neutral stance was anticipated on general grounds in chapter 1, where it was pointed out that differences between the two kinds of medicine were not prejudicial either way. And it can now be seen that two particular differences – and two important differences at that – are not prejudicial. For in recognizing the conceptual importance of 'illness' and of its properties as a value term, the relative prominence of 'mental illness' and the strength of its evaluative connotations are seen to be no more prejudicial to psychological medicine, than the relative prominence of 'physical disease' and the strength of its factual connotations are prejudicial to physical medicine. By virtue of these differences, psychological medicine is conceptually more problematic and hence in this respect clinically more demanding. But that is all.

With respect to the differences between physical medicine and psychological medicine, however, the reverse view of chapter 4 goes further than mere neutrality. For, incomplete as it is, it already provides at least a potential explanation of them. This goes back to the way in which the relationship between the concepts employed in the two kinds of medicine is understood. In the conventional view, 'mental illness' is measured against what is taken to be the paradigm 'physical illness'; hence the differences between them are minimized by the supporters of 'mental illness' and emphasized by its opponents. In a reverse view, on the other hand, it is at least possible that 'mental illness' and 'physical illness' are alike in being subspecies of some (as yet to be defined) general concept of 'illness'. But if this is so, if the 'illness' in the two subspecies is as it were a constant, then the differences between them could be, or could reflect, differences in the properties of their respective constituents – emotions, beliefs and so on in the case of mental illness, feelings and sensations in the case of physical illness. A reverse view thus suggests a quite different approach to understanding the differences between psychological and physical medicine. Moreover, to the extent that this approach succeeds – that is, to the extent that relevant differences are found in the properties of the constituents of the two kinds of illness – the stronger becomes the case for there being a general concept, 'illness', of which 'mental illness' and 'physical illness' are indeed both subspecies.

With these points in mind, then, we will consider in the remainder of this section, two kinds of properties of the constituents of illness, empirical and evaluative. Taking the empirical first, the results of chapter 4 show that the empirical properties of illness constituents are important, if in no other ways, to the development of disease categories. Differences between the empirical properties of mental-illness constituents and those of physical-illness constituents should therefore result in differences between the disease categories developed in psychological medicine and those developed in physical medicine. And this is what is found. Examples of a wide variety of mental illnesses will be considered in chapters 8, 9 and 10. But it can be seen in a general way that, compared with feelings and sensations, the majority of mental-illness constituents tend to be more difficult to describe reliably and have less well-defined associations and less well-understood bodily causes. Compared with physical-illness constituents, therefore, mental-illness constituents are short on just those empirical properties which are necessary for the development of disease categories of the kinds to be found in physical medicine. Hence it is that, compared with these, mental-disease categories are, by and large, difficult to establish in the first place (thus leading to greater variation in the actual categories employed), applied clinically with less reliability, and defined on the whole symptomatically, rather than in terms of their causes. In all these ways, then, as we saw in chapter 4, the clinical utility of mental-disease categories at their present stage of development is less than that of physical-disease categories. And this is one reason for the relative eclipse of the concept of 'mental disease' by that of 'mental illness'.

There is one clear exception to this, albeit an exception which proves the rule. There is a variety of mental-illness constituent, namely, cognitive phenomena (defects in memory, attention and intellect), the empirical properties of which are closer to those of physical illness constituents than those of other mental-illness constituents. Correspondingly, mental illnesses constituted by cognitive phenomena (for example, dementias, amnesias and confusional states) are in many respects closer conceptually to physical illnesses than to other mental illnesses. Thus cognitive phenomena, in so far as they are constituents of mental illness, are, on the whole, relatively easy to diagnose reliably, they are grouped into well-defined syndromes, and their bodily causes are reasonably well understood. It is true that the precise changes in brain function underlying these conditions are not well defined. But it seems at least likely that changes in brain function of some recognizably pathological kind are involved. For cognitive disorders are known to be due to the effects on the brain of relatively gross aetiological agents; agents indeed, such as toxins, traumas and infections which are familiar aetiological agents in physical medicine. In all these respects, then, cognitive changes as mental-illness constituents are similar in their empirical properties to physical-illness constituents. Consequently, cognitive disorders are grouped into well-defined disease categories, many of which include associated features (for example neurological and other signs) and some of which are aetiologically based. And since these categories are as useful clinically as those employed in physical medicine, the concept of 'disease' itself is more or less as prominent in respect of cognitive disorders as it is in physical medicine generally.

Overall, therefore, there is a rough correlation between the empirical properties of illness constituents and the conceptual properties of the illnesses constituted by them, suggesting that the former contribute generally to the latter. However, there must be contributions from other sources as well. There are three reasons for supposing this to be so. The first is one of scale. The differences between mental-illness constituents and physical-illness constituents with regard to their empirical properties are not large enough to explain the extent of the conceptual differences between 'mental illness' and 'physical illness'. Mental-illness constituents are indeed difficult to identify, but, as Wing and others have shown (for example, Wing *et al.*, 1974), they may be reliably identified none the less. Moreover, the reliability with which not only physical-illness constituents (that is, feelings and sensations) but also associated bodily signs (Butterworth and Reppert, 1960) and radiological (Etter *et al.*, 1960) and biochemical (Belk and Sunderman, 1947) test results may be identified is often no greater than that reported for many mental-illness constituents. Reliable identification of the latter requires some training; but then so does the reliable identification of physical-illness constituents and of bodily signs and clinical test results. Furthermore, if causal disease categories figure prominently in physical medicine, symptomatic categories were a necessary precursor of these (cf. chapter 4), and in many instances (for example, migraine and epilepsy) they are still important clinically. Similarly, therefore, in psychological medicine, symptomatic disease categories carry useful implications for prognosis and treatment. Further, as progress is made in the brain sciences, so it may be anticipated that a shift from symptomatic to causal disease categories will occur in psychological medicine, comparable to some extent with that which has already occurred in physical medicine (chapter 2; but see also chapter 12. And we should not forget, of course, that even in the present state of our knowledge, psychological factors may figure in the definitions of HDf2-type physical diseases, e.g., "psychogenic asthma"; and vice versa, e.g., "organic psychosis".)

The second reason is one of distribution. The correlation already noted, between the empirical properties of illness constituents and the conceptual properties of illnesses, holds only for very large clinical groups. If this correlation is looked at in more detail, it breaks down. In particular, as we will see in chapter 10, clinically important conceptual *difficulties* tend to arise in psychological medicine more, rather than less, commonly where empirical difficulties are less, rather than more, in evidence. That is to say, conceptual difficulties tend to arise in psychological medicine where, in the terminology of chapter 1, the condition of the patient as such is not at issue. It is where a patient is known to be anxious or depressed, to hold certain beliefs or to be subject to certain impulses, that clinically important conceptual difficulties about the status of their condition as illness are most likely to arise.

The third reason comes closer still to clinical difficulties. It is that the most important conceptual difference between 'mental illness' and 'physical illness' in relation to clinical difficulties is one that has no obvious connection with the empirical properties of illness constituents at all. The difference in question is the difference in the relative strengths of their evaluative connotations. As noted earlier, it is mainly because the diagnosis of mental illness raises questions of value in ways or to an extent that the diagnosis of physical illness does not, that Szasz and others have claimed that mental illness is not really illness at all. And it is for similar reasons that other authors such as Boorse have sought to eliminate the evaluative connotations of 'mental illness', at least as it is used in technical contexts. But these questions of value and these evaluative connotations are not explained by the empirical properties of the phenomena by which mental illnesses are typically constituted.

This third reason thus suggests a second, quite distinct contribution to the differences between 'mental illness' and 'physical illness', viz. that made by the *evaluative* properties of the phenomena by which they are respectively constituted. On any reverse view these evaluative properties are clearly likely to be important, and it can be seen already from the results of chapters 3 and 4 that in fact they are. Thus, in chapter 3, a mechanism was noted by which the evaluative connotations of value terms can vary with context. These connotations were found to vary inversely with the extent to which the criteria for the value judgements expressed are settled or agreed upon. The less settled the criteria, the more will questions of value tend to be raised by the use of a value term, and hence the stronger will be its evaluative connotations. In chapter 4 this mechanism helped to explain the difference in the strengths of the evaluative connotations of 'illness' and 'disease' in physical medicine. Similarly, as will now be shown, it helps to explain the difference in the strengths of the evaluative connotations of 'mental illness' and 'physical illness'.

Consider anxiety (or fear) as a typical constituent of mental illness, compared with pain as a typical constituent of physical illness. The criteria by which anxiety is evaluated, the kinds or qualities or degrees of anxiety that are evaluated positively or negatively, and the extent of these evaluations, vary far more widely than the corresponding criteria for pain. Anxiety, although commonly unwelcome, can be welcome; even extreme anxiety can be "arousing" or "exciting"; we speak of the "thrill" of fear, of dangerous "sports", of horror films as "entertainment". But pain, even mild pain, is almost invariably (though not quite invariably) unwelcome; for the most part (though not quite always) it is at best a necessary evil; and the extent to which it is negatively evaluated, at least by the person experiencing it, is roughly proportional to its intensity. The variation in question here is not in the capacity to experience anxiety or pain; nor is it in the ability to tolerate these experiences. Rather, it is a variation in the way in which a *given* experience of anxiety or pain is evaluated. And to say that this variation is wider for anxiety than pain is to say that the criteria by which anxiety is evaluated are less settled than the criteria by which pain is evaluated.

It thus follows, from the results of chapter 3, that if 'illness' is a value term, as in any reverse view it is understood to be, then its evaluative connotations will be more marked when it is used in respect of anxiety than when it is used in respect of pain. If a (negative) value judgement is expressed by 'illness', and if the criteria by which anxiety is evaluated are less settled than those by which pain is evaluated, then the judgement as to whether someone who is anxious is ill will be more likely to raise questions of value than the corresponding judgement about someone who is in pain. By extension, then, in so far as mental-illness constituents are in general like anxiety in this respect, while physical-illness constituents are in general like pain, the judgement as to whether someone is mentally ill will be more likely to raise questions of value than the corresponding judgement as to whether someone is physically ill. In other words (and this brings us back to clinical problems) the *diagnosis* of mental illness will be more likely to raise questions of value than the diagnosis of physical illness. Hence, although – indeed *because* – 'mental illness' and 'physical illness' are both value terms, the evaluative connotations of 'mental illness' in clinical practice will be more marked than those of 'physical illness'.

In this way, then, differences between the evaluative properties of mental-illness constituents and physical-illness constituents make an important contribution to the conceptual differences between psychological medicine and physical medicine, and one which is *prima facie* directly relevant to the clinically more problematic nature of 'mental illness'. These properties also contribute in other ways. They contribute, for example, to the relative variability of 'mental illness' compared with 'physical illness'. Both concepts vary in their denotation, cross-culturally and historically. But 'mental illness' is more variable in these respects than 'physical illness', and this could clearly be a reflection of the greater variation in the criteria by which typical mental-illness constituents are evaluated (Reznek, 1987, Ch. 1, reviews a number of examples showing the variable denotation of physical-disease concepts). Then again, these properties contribute to the relative prominence of 'mental illness' compared with 'mental disease' in psychological medicine – for to say that there is relatively wide variation in the evaluative criteria for the constituents of mental illness is just another way of saying that in relation to mental illness relatively few conditions will fall into the subcategory, Id, of conditions widely regarded as illnesses; and it is from this subcategory, according to the argument of chapter 4, that the concept of 'disease' arises. All in all, then, the evaluative properties of mental-illness constituents are important here, very much as would be expected in a reverse-view analysis of the medical concepts.

The starting point for this discussion of the conceptual differences between psychological medicine and physical medicine was the observation that the essentially neutral attitude towards these differences first taken up in chapter 1 was fully justified. The explanation now given for these differences provides further justification for this attitude. For if these differences are derived from differences in the properties, empirical and evaluative, of the phenomena by which mental illness and physical illness are respectively constituted, then the concept of 'mental illness' is no more prejudiced by the differences between it and 'physical illness' than is the concept of 'physical illness'. Thus, against Szasz-style objections to the concept of 'mental illness', the present analysis suggests that in so far as both 'physical illness' and 'mental illness' faithfully *reflect* the properties of their respective illness constituents, both are *endorsed* by the differences between them. 'Mental illness', in being the *more* value-laden of the two, is as sound conceptually as 'physical illness' is sound in being the *less* value-laden. The point is similar to, and reinforces, that made at the start of this section about the relative prominence of 'illness' and 'disease' themselves in psychological and physical medicine. That 'mental illness' is the more value-laden makes it the more difficult concept to work with clinically. But it is no less sound a concept for that.

As judged against requirement 2, therefore, perhaps more so even than requirement 1, the reverse-view analysis developed in chapter 4 is seen to have made good progress towards our target problems, the non-empirical problems of clinical practice. Even now, though, we are not yet quite ready to tackle these problems. For we have not yet examined a sufficiently wide range of mental-illness constituents to be able to say that anxiety really is typical of mental-illness constituents generally. Indeed, in the required respect, in the variability of the criteria by which it is evaluated, it could well be that it is not typical at all. Depression, another common mental-illness constituent, is probably similar to anxiety in this respect. But what of the symptoms of, say, schizophrenia; namely, delusions, hallucinations and so on (described in detail in chapter 10)? Schizophrenia, surely, is a condition which is negatively evaluated as consistently as, say, coronary thrombosis: in the study by Campbell *et al.* (1979) of the attribution of 'disease', these two conditions came out almost equal; and both scored substantially higher than depression. The particular kind of value which is expressed by the medical concepts may be important generally in medicine (Gillon, 1986). But in relation to psychological medicine, and with our target problems in mind, it is inescapably so. For the issue raised by schizophrenia, in the debate about 'mental illness' at least, is not so much whether it is a *bad* condition as whether it is a bad condition of the *particular* kind which is properly thought of as illness. It is this issue, similarly, which is at the heart of many other clinically important conceptual problems. Is the psychopath, in the well-worn phrase, mad or bad? Or the alcoholic? Or the hysteric? And if mad, is madness an illness?

It is to this issue, then, to the particular *kind* of negative value that is expressed by 'illness', and hence to a more complete analysis of the concept itself, that we must now turn.

ILLNESS AND DISEASE
AS MEDICAL VALUE TERMS

Part III

Part III

6

Dysfunction and function

Any study of the particular kind of value which is expressed by 'illness', if it is to be at all comprehensive, must include some consideration at least, of the particular kind of value which is expressed by 'dysfunction'; for the two kinds of value are so closely linked. As shown generally in chapter 4, they are linked, first, as the concepts of 'illness' and 'dysfunction' themselves are linked – for example, as cause and effect by way of 'disease', and, elsewhere, in being used sometimes of the same conditions. Then they are linked, too, in their own right, the value judgement expressed by 'dysfunction' being derived in part at least from that which is expressed by 'illness'; and the two value judgements being similar to the extent that both are negative value judgements distinct from, e.g., negative aesthetic and moral value judgements.

Given the existence of these close links, there is in the present study a more or less direct obligation in investigating one to investigate the other. For the links between them are themselves important features of ordinary usage, which, under our first outcome criterion, stand to be explained. And all the more so because, notwithstanding the links between them, the two kinds of value judgement are none the less distinct. They are distinct, first, as 'illness' and 'dysfunction' are distinct, *as* cause and effect (see chapter 4), and, where they are used of the same condition, in that the subjects to which they refer are different (in the example in chapter 4 it is the person's legs which are not functioning properly but the person himself who is ill). Then again, there are many negatively evaluated functional conditions of bodies (let alone of machines) which are not directly related to 'illness' at all: the condition of being disabled, for example, or that of being wounded or just plain unfit (chapter 2). Under our first outcome criterion, therefore, the differences

89

(as well as the similarities) between illness and each of these dysfunctional bodily conditions, as well as that of disease, stand to be explained, as indeed stand to be explained the differences between all these conditions, illness included, and conditions such as sleep and death.

There are, then, a number of good, if rather general, reasons for enlarging the scope of the present section to include the concept of 'dysfunction' as well as that of 'illness', and to encompass the value judgements expressed by both concepts. But there is also a further, more specific reason, a reason arising directly from the results set out in the last three chapters, or rather from the gaps in these results. For the particular gap which is the starting point for this section, the inability at the end of chapter 5 to explain fully the evaluative properties of 'mental illness', is closely related to certain gaps in the results for 'dysfunction' and 'disease' in chapters 3 and 4. If any one of these gaps is to be closed, therefore, it is likely that all of them will have to be. Thus, the assumption at the start of chapter 4 that 'illness' is a value term, was prompted, merely, by the conclusion of chapter 3, that 'dysfunction' is a value term. But although this assumption was largely borne out by the results of chapters 4 and 5, no actual connection was drawn between the two concepts. And this omission, together with the failure in chapter 5 to explain the evaluative properties of 'mental illness', might put in doubt not only the assumption of chapter 4, that 'illness' is a value term, but also, by association, the conclusion of chapter 3 that 'dysfunction' is a value term.

To this extent, then, the whole of the argument of chapters 3–5 stands or falls as a piece. Hence, in pursuing the main objective of this section, the characterization of the particular kind of value which is expressed by 'illness', much the same ground has to be covered as before: from "dysfunction", therefore, in the present chapter, to 'illness' in chapter 7 and so back to 'mental illness' in chapter 8.

A descriptivist reviewing the debate presented in chapter 3 might be inclined to argue that the issues raised in passing from non-functional to functional objects (specifically, from straw-berries to bodily parts and organs) were too lightly set aside.

And certainly the non-descriptivist argument, as presented in that debate, was far from conclusive in respect of the latter; for it relied on only one, and on one possibly atypical, example, that of kidneys.

Thus, it was conceded to descriptivism that for functional as opposed to non-functional objects there are logical, not merely psychological, limits to the criteria by which they may be evaluated, positively or negatively – that is to say, limits set by the very functions by which such objects, as functional objects, are defined. But it was denied that the non-descriptivist principle, "no ought from an is", was thereby impaired. For it was argued that the functions of functional objects could not themselves be defined value-free. And it was here that kidneys were introduced by way of example. Yet it is here, too, that kidneys are atypical. For it may well be true, as was claimed, that in order to define 'kidney' in terms of kidney function, and in order, therefore, to set a logical limit to the criteria by which kidney functioning may be evaluated, it is necessary to introduce the value term 'waste'. But there would seem to be no counterparts to 'waste' in respect of a large majority of other organs and bodily parts: hearts just pump blood, eyes see, hands grip and manipulate, and so on. In respect of this large majority of organs and bodily parts, therefore, a descriptivist account of their evaluation, and of the evaluation of their functioning would appear to be possible.

This further descriptivist argument, used in respect of bodily parts and organs, is apparently borne out by analogy with non-biological functional objects. Indeed, use is often made of such an analogy in the literature, as by Boorse (1975, p. 59), who points out that the way in which the functioning of bodily parts and organs is evaluated is conceptually similar, at least in technical contexts, to the way in which the functioning of, say, machines is evaluated. But the evaluation of machine functioning, it is claimed, is based on purely factual considerations, so that here an 'ought' really would seem to be derived from an 'is'. There would thus seem to be a good *prima-facie* case for the same to be true of the evaluation in technical contexts of bodily parts and organs.

It is with this analogy between biological and non-biological functional objects that we will be concerned in this chapter. We will address three questions: first, and at greatest length, whether, and if so precisely how, non-biological functional objects are defined in terms of their functions; second, whether, and if so precisely why, limits are thereby set to the criteria by which the functioning of such objects may be evaluated; and third, whether, and if so whether in support or denial of descriptivism, similar limits are set to the criteria by which the functioning of biological functional objects may be evaluated.

Non-biological functional objects

A functional object, whether biological or non–biological, is an object with a function. The function of a functional object is that which it does in functioning. In order to define 'functional object' in terms of 'function', therefore, the concept of 'functioning' must first be defined.

Consider a car. What is it for a car to be functioning? Well, it would seem, at least, that for a car to be functioning it must indeed be (as has just been implied) *doing* something – doing something, that is to say, as distinct from something being done or happening to it. A car travelling along under its own power is functioning; the car itself is doing something. But a car being towed along or transported on a lorry is not functioning; rather, something is being done or is happening to it. By this, however, is begged the question of the meaning in this context of the word 'do'. For not all doings are functional doings, as it were. A specification is thus required of 'functional doing'.

Functional doing must first be understood to include things done in or by not moving as well as things done in or by moving. It is true, of course, that since most functional objects function in or by moving, functioning objects are usually moving objects. But not all functional objects function in this active way. It is in *not* moving, for example, that doorstops and paperweights function. Doorstops and paper weights just sit there. This is what they do. Moreover, it is in this stationary sense of 'doing' that, say, a car's brakes function. Brakes, like engines, have to be put into use. But once in use, brakes, unlike engines, function in *not* moving.

Not moving and moving are thus both species of functional doing. Yet as a specification of 'functional doing', "moving and/or not moving" is too broad. For in this sense of 'doing', non-functional as well as functional objects do things, as distinct from having things done and from things happening to them. A boulder rolls down a hillside, or, it is rolled. A boulder sits on a hillside, or, it is wedged there. Further, in this sense of 'doing', functional objects themselves, by virtue of what Hempel (1965) has called their "adventitious properties", may do things which are coincidental or even contrary to the things which they do in functioning. Cars with their brakes left off roll down hillsides, for example; so do suitably shaped doorstops and paperweights. And cars with no petrol in them just sit there.

But here at least, it may seem, the difference is obvious enough: namely, that that which a functional object does in functioning is that which it was designed to do. A car is designed to move about by the action of its engine and to stop and keep still by the action of its brakes. And to these things which it does in functioning, its rolling down hills when its brakes have been left off and its just sitting there when it has no petrol are (at best) coincidental. By contrast, just sitting there is precisely what a doorstop or a paperweight *is* designed to do. While as to non-functional objects, like boulders on hillsides, these, *ex hypothesi*, are not designed to do anything at all.

Yet as a specification of 'functional doing', this is now not too broad but too narrow. For while it is surely true that functional doing is the doing by a functional object of that which it was designed to do, 'that which it was designed to do' is not specified sufficiently by a description merely of the movings or not movings of the object in question. Such a description is necessary, certainly: one could not (ordinarily) be said to know what a car was designed to do unless one knew at least that it was designed to move about by the action of an engine and to stop and keep still by the action of a brake. But this is not sufficient. For one could not (ordinarily) be said to know what a car was designed to do unless one knew also the purpose, the particular purpose which, by its movings or not movings, it was designed to serve – namely, that of carrying people and things. Otherwise it might be a bulldozer or an army tank, say. Generalizing, therefore, that which a functional object was designed to do, and hence that which it actually does in functioning, is not just to perform certain movings or not movings, but, therein and/or thereby, to serve some particular purpose.

The specification of 'functional doing' is therefore a two-part specification. It is a specification involving not only the mechanism but also the purpose, not only the means but also the ends, of a functional object. Interestingly, the words 'function' and 'functioning', although often implying both parts of this specification, are none the less sometimes used with only one or the other part mainly in mind – as when one asks of a functional object, on the one hand, "What is its function?" meaning "What is its purpose?", or, on the other, "How does it function?" meaning "How does it serve that purpose?"; or when a car engine, being test-run in a garage, is said to be functioning even though, at the time, it is being run for the purpose of testing it, not for the purpose of driving a car. But these as it were part uses of 'function' and 'functioning', in preference to the use of other words or phrases from the "purpose/means and ends" stable, arise only in respect of functional objects. They are thus both logically dependent on (their meaning being derived from), and in turn imply, their full two-part uses defined by the specification of 'functional doing' here derived.

'Functional doing' is thus purposeful doing. And once this idea, of the 'designed for' purpose of a functional object, is introduced, a number of loose ends implicit in what has been said thus far about 'functional doing' can be tidied up. A first loose end, working backwards, is in the distinction drawn a moment ago between those movings/not movings of a functional object which are functional and those which are adventitious. It was said, rightly, that that which a functional object does in functioning is that which it was designed to do. But if "that which it was designed to do" were limited just to the movings/not movings of the object in question (as on p. 93, strictly speaking, it *was* limited), then, as a device for distinguishing the functional from the adventitious of these movings/not movings, it would have been ineffective. For without the idea of purpose, of the object in question's "designed-for" purpose, 'that which it was designed to do' would mean only "that which is a product or result of its design". And in this purpose-free sense, the adventitious, as well as the functional, movings/not movings of a functional object are products or outcomes of its design. In this purpose-free sense, a car's rolling down hills when its brakes have been left off and its just sitting there when it has no petrol are as much things which it is designed to do – they are as much products or outcomes of its design – as are its moving about by the action of its engine and its stopping and keeping still by the action of its brakes. Indeed, in this purpose-free sense, a car's emission of carbon monoxide and its smearing of rubber on roads are as much things which it is designed to do – they are as much products or outcomes of its design – as are its carrying of people or things.

A second loose end, still working backwards, lies in the claim, made with reference to doorstops and paperweights, that not moving is as much a species of functional doing as moving. In the form in which it was made, the precise sense in which this claim is true was not made clear. Indeed, with the subsequent suggestion that the sense in question might be similar to that in which non-functional objcts (like boulders on hillsides) do things in not moving, it might be thought that the claim itself was too strongly made. For, it might be said, non-functional objects at least, when they are *not* moving, are not really *doing* things in quite the same clear sense in which they are doing things when they are moving. To this extent, therefore, not moving, though perhaps the equal of moving as a species of functional doing, is not quite its equal as a species of non-functional doing. There is, no doubt, *some* sense in which, by contrast with things which are done or happen to them, non-functional objects may be said to do things in not moving. The boulder just sitting on a hillside, in the example given earlier, might (possibly) be said to be doing something compared with one which is wedged there. But then, compared with the boulder which is rolling down the hillside, the boulder sitting there would surely be said not to be doing anything at all. And what, really, is it doing? It is indeed just sitting there. It is here, then, that this loose end is now ready to be tidied up.

For, as can now be seen, "just" sitting there is what doorstops and paperweights, in functioning, are *not* doing. These, too, in functioning, sit there. But in functioning they are not *just* sitting there. For in functioning, they are serving the purposes they were designed to serve, holding doors back and papers down respectively.

It is in this purpose-serving sense, therefore, that not moving is as much a species of functional doing as moving. And in recognizing this, the way is cleared for tidying up a third loose end – namely, that although it is true, as was claimed earlier, that not moving and moving are (in the sense now clarified) equally species of functional doing, it is not true, as was perhaps implied, that there are no other species of functional doing than these. For clearly, if functional doing is purposeful doing, functional objects may function not only by moving and not moving but also by whatever is a means to the ends served by them. The ends served by the functional objects so far considered – cars, doorstops and paperweights – are ends either of moving things or of keeping things still; and correspondingly, the means by which such objects function are their properties of being mobile or immobile. But lights function – that is, they light things – by being luminous; heaters heat things by being hot; pillows cushion things by being soft; knives cut things by being sharp; and so on. Movement, of course, even where it is not directly involved in the functioning of a functional object, is often contingently necessary none the less – lights have to be switched on, and so on. Indeed, physics tells us that all the properties of objects, not just their properties of mobility and immobility, are products of the movements of their components, of their atomic and subatomic structures, and of the force carrying particles by which these structures are maintained. All the same, it is in the world of everyday experience that objects function; in everyday experience objects have properties other than just those of mobility and immobility; and in everyday experience objects may function – they may serve the purposes they were designed to serve – by means of any kind of property whatsoever.

This leads to a fourth and final loose end, in the very distinction from which the present analysis of 'functioning' began. In discussing cars, it was said that for a functional object to be functioning it must at least be doing something as distinct from something being done or happening to it. And, as we have *now* come to understand 'functional doing', this was right enough; to be functioning a functional object must be serving (or doing that which is directed towards serving) the purpose it was designed to serve. But as 'functional doing' was understood on p. 92, before the introduction of the idea of purpose, in terms only of the purpose-free pushings and pullings to which non-functional as well as functional objects are subject, it would not have been right at all. It would have been right up to a point, perhaps, for objects like motor cars which do indeed function by moving as distinct from being moved. A car, as was said, serves the purpose it was designed to serve (that of carrying people and things) by travelling along under its own power, as distinct from being towed or transported. But what of a car trailer, say? This, on the contrary, serves the same purpose as a car (carrying people and things), but by *being* towed. In the purpose-free, non-functional sense of 'doing', therefore, for a trailer to be functioning, far from the trailer doing something, something must be being done to it. The original distinction thus stands, but only with respect to 'functional doing' as it is now (properly) understood – that is, as purpose*ful* doing.

The "designed for" purpose of a functional object is thus wound inextricably into the concept of 'functional doing'. It distinguishes functional from adventitious movings/not movings (and other properties) of functional objects; it underlies the sense in which not-moving, or any other property of a functional object, may be as much a species of functional doing as moving; and it provides the key to the sense in which functional doing is any kind of *doing* at all. Indeed, it is itself a mark of just how inextricably the idea of the "designed-for" purpose of a functional object is wound into the concept of 'functional doing', that before it was introduced all these loose ends were only implicit in the argument. For although up to that point the sense of 'functional doing', as specified, was (strictly speaking) a purpose-free sense, so crucial is the "designed-for" purpose of a functional object to the *actual* sense of this notion that, even before it was introduced explicitly, it was already there, in the background as it were, implicitly or unconsciously there, and thus available covertly to serve the argument as it developed.

Not, though, that the "designed-for" means by which a functional object functions, should thus be considered any the less significant conceptually. As already emphasized both means and ends are necessary to the sense of 'functional doing'. After all, for any particular "designed-for" purpose, there will often be a number of different means by which that purpose could be served. And for a functional object to be functioning, not only must it be serving its particular "designed-for" purpose, it must be serving that purpose by its particular "designed-for" means: a car, even if it is carrying people and things, is not functioning if it is being towed or transported. Thus a specification of 'functional doing' must indeed be a two-part specification; that which a functional object does in functioning being to serve (or attempt to serve) the purpose it was designed to serve by the means by which it was designed to serve it.

Turning now to the notion of 'functional object', it is easily seen that the same two-part specification is necessary. A doorstop, for example, is an object designed for the purpose of stopping doors by means of weighting − not, for example, hooking − them back. Whereas a paperweight, which might otherwise be identical to a doorstop, is an object designed for the purpose of keeping papers tidy by means of weighting (not, for example, pinning) them down. And 'motor car', in the *Shorter Oxford English Dictionary*, is actually defined as "a carriage ..." (= its "designed-for" purpose) "... propelled by a motor" (= its "designed-for" means).

With 'functional object', however, the importance of the "designed-for" part of the specification is further emphasized. For it is by this that a functional object, being an object designed to serve a particular purpose by a particular means, is marked out from an object merely *used* to serve a particular purpose by a particular means. Any object, after all, functional or not, may in principle be used to serve a wide range of purposes (logically, perhaps, any purpose, though of course not any purpose successfully). But for an object to be a functional object – and thus for it to be capable, at least, of functioning – it must be *designed* to serve a particular purpose (even if that purpose is very widely defined, e.g., as in 'all-purpose camping tool'). The extent of this "design" varies, of course. Some functional objects are no more than selected natural objects: sling shots, for example, are just selected stones. Then again, in respect of such objects there may be some ambiguity as to whether they are objects merely used to serve particular purposes by particular means, or whether they are, as such, functional objects. A boulder brought home from a hillside for the purpose of stopping doors may be thought of either *as* a doorstop or as a boulder being *used* as a doorstop. More often, though, functional objects are not just selected. Usually, by processes of greater or lesser complexity, they are made. In which case, since that which is made, the actual object constructed, is defined by the intentions of its designer, even the possibility of ambiguity is removed.

Evaluation of non-biological functional objects

Consider cars again. What is it for a car not to be functioning properly? Clearly, since cars function in moving and keeping still, their state of motion must somehow come into judgements about whether they are functioning properly. What is crucial, however, equally for 'not functioning properly' as for 'functioning', is not the state of motion of a car as such, but its attribution. The notion that a car is *not* functioning properly, like that of it functioning properly, involves the idea that its state of motion is in some sense something it, the car itself, is doing, as distinct from something that is being done or is happening to it. And this is true even of atypical states of motion. Swerving movements, for example, are atypical of cars – that is of ordinary cars on ordinary roads. And a car which is swerving may be not functioning properly. But a swerving car which is not functioning properly has to be distinguished from one to which something is being done (for example, one which is being driven badly) or one to which something is happening (for example, it is skidding on a patch of ice). In the case of 'not functioning properly', furthermore, it is immediately clear that the sense of 'do' implied by this distinction must be such as to cover not moving as well as moving. For the (perhaps) paradigm case of a car not functioning properly is the car that won't start. And here, too, the distinction between 'doing' and 'done/happens to' is apparent. For the car that is not functioning properly in not starting is to be distinguished from one that is being started in the wrong way (as in "flooding the carburettor", for example) or indeed from one which has simply not been switched on. This latter case, incidentally, brings out the point that just as 'functioning' must cover not moving as well as moving, so 'not functioning properly' must cover moving as well as not moving. For the car that (in the empirically unlikely case) bursts into life when it has not been switched on, as much as the car that won't start, is not functioning properly.

'Functional doing' is thus central to the concept of 'not functioning properly', as it is to that of 'functioning'. And in the case of cars at least, an intuitively natural way to mark out the sense of 'functional doing' in relation to 'not functioning properly', is by bringing in the notion of something mechanically wrong; for example, jammed brakes or steering failure in the case of a car swerving, and a flat battery in the case of the car that won't start. Nor is this, on the face of it, merely tautologous. Mechanical failure, it is true, is itself a case of a functional object – in this case one or other of the *parts* of the car concerned – not functioning properly. But the question of whether a part of a car is functioning properly could normally be settled by reference to the manufacturer's specification. Of course, for this way of settling the question to be effective, the specification would have to be more than a mere blueprint of the parts of the car; for it is the operation of these parts which is material. But it would have to be more, even, than an operational manual, of the kind used by a garage mechanic. Such a specification, showing *how* the car in question functions, is certainly necessary. Too many or too radical departures from this will result in a car of a different type, or even in a machine which is not a car at all. But within these limits, the functioning of a part, though different from that specified (in the manual) might be more or less or equally satisfactory. Indeed, a substitute part, though a different part altogether from the original, might function as well or better. Similarly, even though all the parts of a car function according to their design, the car itself will not function properly if that design is faulty. Of course, there are circumstances in which an individual part may fail to function properly without the car itself breaking down, as with a fail-safe back-up system. The point to be taken, rather, is the logical point, that in order to distinguish good from bad functioning by reference to the original design specification, it is necessary that there be included in that specification descriptions not only of *how* the car is intended to function – that is, of its mechanism – but also of what the car as a whole is intended to do *in* functioning – that is, of its "designed-for" purpose. The latter description may be more or less detailed, more or less explicit, but it must be there. For it is according to the success with which a car does that which it was designed to do that its functioning, and hence the functioning of its parts, is evaluated.

The argument by which the two-part specification (first of 'functioning' and then of 'functional object') was reached in the last subsection has now in effect been recapitulated. Inherent in the idea of a car not functioning properly is the distinction by which functioning itself is marked out – namely, that between things the car itself does and things that are done or happen to it. The relevant sense of 'do', however, is one which in principle covers any state of motion of a car, whether moving or keeping still. In the case of a car not functioning properly the intuitively natural way to mark out this sense of 'do', is by reference to mechanical failure, to the idea of some part of the car in question not functioning properly, which in turn is referred to the car's design specification. However, as for 'functioning' so now for 'not functioning properly', the required design specification must include descriptions not only of *how* the car in question is intended to function (its "designed-for" mechanism) but also of what it is intended to do *in* functioning (its "designed-for" purpose). Moreover, the recapitulation can be taken further. For as will now be clear, the analysis of 'not functioning properly' can be extended, as that of 'functioning' was extended, to functional objects of other kinds (in particular to non-mechanical functional objects), and so as to bring out the significance of the distinction between a functional object's "designed-for" purpose and other purposes for which it might be used (a car's functioning is not to be judged by its efficacy as a bulldozer, for example). Interestingly, the negative case, that of 'not functioning properly', here suggests a further insight into the notion of a "designed-for" purpose, and hence into that of 'functional' doing. We will return to the importance of negative cases generally in analysis in chapter 12. What is shown by the negative case here, though, is that the "designed-for" purpose of a functional object must include some idea of the circumstances in which the object in question is expected to function. A car skidding on a patch of ice is a car to which something is happening. A "snow cat" skidding on the other hand, being a vehicle designed for the purpose of transporting people and things but in arctic conditions, would be not functioning properly.

So the argument of the present subsection recapitulates, and to some degree extends, the argument of the last. And the significance of this is that the information necessary, *all* the information necessary, to judge whether a swerving car is functioning properly, is contained in the (two-part) design specification by which the car itself is defined. And from this it follows, consistently with the descriptivist view, that to know what a car *is* is also to know what it is for a car to be functioning *properly*. Not completely, perhaps, since there may be aspects of a car's functioning – certain kinds of aesthetic aspect, for example – which are not covered by its design specification; as when a preference is expressed for a certain quality of engine noise, say. Some, indeed, might seek to draw a distinction here between 'functioning properly' and 'functioning well', arguing that, strictly speaking, it is only the criteria for 'functioning properly' which are determined by a given car's design specification, and hence by what that car is. On the other hand, though, a particular kind of engine noise could be, and in sports cars often is, part of the design specification. So that, consistently with the general line of argument which is now developing, those aesthetic aspects of a car's functioning which are genuinely *not* part of its design specification are perhaps more correctly thought of as having nothing to do with its functioning, either properly or well. All the same, the essential descriptivist conclusion would remain: namely, that there is a definite logical limit to the criteria by which a car's functioning may be evaluated, a limit set by the (two-part, functional) definition of 'car'. And this conclusion, generalized to non-biological functional objects as a whole, thus provides support for the "further" descriptivist argument with which this chapter is concerned.

Biological functional objects

What are the implications of this analysis of non-biological functional objects for a descriptivist account of biological functional objects? First, on the debit side, the inadequacy of what might now be called non-specific descriptivism, is underscored. A statistical account, for example, of the kind mentioned in chapter 2, when applied to the present example of a car swerving, would have entirely failed to distinguish cases of the car not functioning properly from cases in which something was being done or was happening to it. For in all three kinds of case the (swerving) movements of the car, although statistically atypical, were the same. Moreover, there are further cases in which there would be nothing wrong at all with a car moving in just this way. Thus, a car put deliberately into a swerve to avoid an accident – or indeed skidding on an icy road – might actually be said to have "handled well". Then again, a reductionist account of the car swerving, an account in which the evaluation of the car's functioning is reduced to an evaluation of the functioning of its parts, would also have failed. For in this case, what counted as a part of the car not functioning properly – that is what counted as mechanical failure – was determined by reference to the "designed-for" purpose of the car as a whole, not vice versa. This last observation, by the way, is obviously relevant to the way in which the relationship between 'disease' and 'illness' is understood, in that it lends support to the idea developed in chapter 4, that what counts as disease is determined by what counts as illness, not vice versa.

On the credit side, though, the adequacy of the further,

more specific, descriptivist argument outlined at the start of this chapter is (on the face of it) endorsed. Indeed, in the preceding two subsections, this argument has effectively been unpacked, showing not only that, but also why, it works. The argument as presented at the start of this chapter, and in chapter 3, was to the effect that since functional objects are defined by their functions, there is a definite logical limit to the criteria by which such objects may be evaluated. And the analysis of the last two subsections now shows that this limit-setting property of the concept of 'function' is derived from the "designed-for" purpose by which, together with a "designed-for" means, functional objects are actually defined. A functional object functions properly to the extent that in what it does *in* functioning, it serves the purpose it was designed to serve. Moreover, the discussion a moment ago of 'functioning properly' and 'functioning well', suggests that a move has already been made towards the main objective of this section – namely, the delineation of the particular kind of value which is expressed by the medical concepts. For the kind of value which is expressed by 'functioning properly' – and possibly also by 'functioning well' – was distinguished in that discussion from aesthetic value. But medical value, as was pointed out at the start of this chapter, is also distinguished from, *inter alia*, aesthetic value. Hence the kind of value which is expressed by 'not functioning properly', as analysed in this section, turns out to be, at least in this respect, similar to the kind of value which is expressed by 'illness'.

The analysis thus shows promise. Yet, as a specifically descriptivist analysis, there is a certain untidiness left over in the move from non-biological to biological functional objects. These two kinds of object, it is true, are in many ways similar. In particular, the crucial descriptivist step, the step from 'is' to 'ought', is available as much for biological as for non-biological functional objects. Biological functional objects, like non-biological, are designed to serve particular purposes; and the criteria by which biological functional objects are judged to be functioning properly may thus be derived, as the corresponding criteria for non-biological functional objects are derived, from the "designed-for" purposes by which they are in part defined.

However, biological functional objects differ from non-biological functional objects in not having designers; biological functional objects, though designed to serve particular purposes in particular ways, are evolved not invented, grown not made. Yet according to the present analysis, it is by reference to the intentions of their designers that the "designed-for" purposes of non-biological functional objects are determined.

Still, this untidiness, it may seem, is easily enough resolved by an obvious extension of the analogy. For, it may be said, are not biological functional objects in this respect like non-biological functional objects the designers of which are no longer extant; like objects recovered from an archaeological dig? In the absence of pictorial or other records, the designers of such objects are not available to arbitrate on the purposes the objects were designed to serve. Yet, where these purposes are not self-evident, they may often be established, if not with certainty at least with a high degree of probability, from a description of the properties of the objects themselves, together at least with reasonable assumptions about the purposes of the people by whom they were designed. As, indeed, the purposes which such objects were designed to serve regularly *are* established by archaeologists. And as, similarly, the purposes which biological functional objects are designed to serve, where these are not self-evident, regularly *are* established by biologists.

Examined more closely, however, this extension of the analogy leaves the move from non-biological to biological functional objects more untidy still. For with its "reasonable assumptions", about the purposes of the people by whom archaeological artefacts were designed, is introduced a (from the point of view of descriptivism) disquieting echo of the argument of chapter 3. In chapter 3, similar "reasonable assumptions", though in that case about the criteria for value judgements, were rejected as the basis for a descriptivist account of 'dysfunction'; because, as was pointed out, however reasonable such assumptions might be, they could provide only a contingent, and not the required logical, link between description and evaluation. Such assumptions, that is to say, were found to connect description and evaluation at most by ordinary, rather than by the required strict, implication. And here, in chapter 6, in the argument by analogy from non-biological to biological functional objects, we find "reasonable assumptions" cropping up again – about purposes, it is true, not values, but serving a similar analytical end, linking description with . . . well, with what?

For now, rather as the appearance of a visual illusion, when one's attention is drawn to some particular feature of it, may suddenly and as a whole begin to shift and change, so, suddenly and as a whole, the appearance of the concept of 'purpose' has begun to shift and change. No longer can it be seen straight-forwardly as a factual concept, as a concern – at least in technical contexts – of engineers, biologists and their (scientific) like. Suddenly, 'purpose' itself appears as an evaluative concept. This is neither a new nor an uncontentious idea (Ans-combe, 1956/7). It indeed raises many of the issues explored in chapter 3 in relation to the is–ought debate. But by one test, at least, that of "non-contradiction" (M. Warnock, 1978, Ch. 3), 'purpose' clearly *is* an evaluative concept. We can see this if we compare the present case with that of, say, 'bitch' and 'female dog'. Here the logical connection clearly is one of strict entailment; and correspondingly it is self-contradictory to describe an animal as a female dog while at the same time denying that it is a bitch. Similarly, then, for 'purpose' and evaluation: to describe something as one's purpose while at the same time denying that one evaluates it (in some sense and *mutatis mutandis*) positively would indeed be self-contradictory. Hence evaluation is *prima facie* strictly entailed by 'purpose', it is part of the very meaning of the term.

There have been hints of this all along, of course; notably in Hempel's distinction between the functional and adventitious properties of a functional object. The essential descriptivist difficulty there was that no description of the properties of a functional object, however complete, could in itself provide for this distinction. So that, just as in chapter 3 in order to get a value judgement out of a statement about something a value judgement had first to be put in, so here, in chapter 6, in order to get a purpose out of a statement about something (in other words, in order for some property of an object to be said to be a functional – that is, a purpose-serving – property) a *purpose* had first to be put in. However, as long as it is only non-biological functional objects that are considered, there is a particular barrier to recognizing that the descriptivist difficulty with 'purpose' (as in this chapter) might be just a special case of the descriptivist difficulty with value judgements generally (in chapter 3). For in the case of non-biological functional objects the necessary 'purpose' is put in – logically, not merely psychologically, put in – by such objects being actually defined by the (in principle) determinate intentions of their designers. The logical, though not always psychological, indeterminacy which is both implicit in and an important signpost to the independence of description and evaluation, is thus, in the case of non-biological functional objects, largely avoided. But it is avoided by introducing (covertly in the concept of 'purpose') an evaluative logical element, rather than, as required by descriptivism, by reducing evaluation to description.

Something along the same lines is true also of biological functional objects. As already emphasized, there are differences. Biological functional objects – hands, hearts and so on – do not have designers. Yet they have "designed-for" purposes. Where do these come from? How do they get into the definitions of what such objects are? Further exploration of the analogy between these and non-biological functional objects would be one way to follow up questions of this kind. Certainly the analogy allows some interesting philosophical slides, for example, 'robot's hand' – 'prosthetic hand (mechanical)' – 'prosthetic hand (biological)' – 'person's hand'. And in the next chapter slides of this kind, together with certain further considerations, will suggest an important logical link between the concept of 'function' (used of objects) and that of 'action' (used of persons). But it can be seen already in a general way, that although the purposes of people (and other organisms) are not limited in the way that those of functional objects are limited, by definition of what they are, none the less there are *some* purposes they would be hard pressed to do without; notably those related to biological needs. Such purposes, although as it were logically optional, are not biologically so. They are therefore *prima facie* well suited to the role of "designed-for" purposes (whatever may be the exact logical mechanism by which they come to fill that role). Not, though, that this lets in a descriptivist account of the evaluation of the functioning of biological functional objects, even in principle. The essential point in this section is that what lies behind the marking out of this or that property of a functional object *as* its purpose is, *inter alia*, the idea that that property is positively evaluated (though of course not necessarily by oneself). And the arguments of chapter 3 show that taking this positive evaluation back even to such general biological needs as survival and/or re-production fails to achieve the descriptivist's objective of deriving evaluative conclusions from descriptive premises alone.

Still, this section is not intended to stand on its own as an account of 'biological functioning'. The point for now is the more limited one that the analogy between biological and non-biological functional objects, pursued as it has been in this chapter on behalf of descriptivism, backfires. For in unpacking the concept of 'function' in respect of non-biological functional objects, it is found that the functioning of such objects cannot be defined value-free after all. And if this is so for non-biological functional objects, objects which Boorse and others regard as paradigmatically suited to analysis along descriptivist lines, then it is even more likely to be so for biological functional objects. Indeed, one point at least is now clear from this analogy: namely, that if 'kidney' is atypical of biological functional objects (as was claimed on behalf of descriptivism at the start of the chapter), then it is so only to the extent that the value judgement 'waste' implicit in the definition of its function, is more explicit than most. Hands do indeed just "grip and manipulate". But the analogy with non-biological functional objects, as now unpacked in this chapter, shows that their gripping and manipulating is marked out from among their other properties as their *purpose*, by (at some logical remove, to be sure) a positive value judgement. There is thus no profit for descriptivism in the analogy between biological and non-biological functional objects. For the conclusion to be drawn from this analogy is that such logical constraints as are placed on the evaluation of functional objects by their being defined in terms of their functions, are, after all, evaluative and not descriptive in origin.

7
Illness and action

Much of what has been said so far about 'illness' has been of a rather general nature. Thus, in chapter 2 a use of 'illness' in which it is distinct in meaning from 'disease' was simply noted; in chapter 4, 'illness', in this use, was shown to be the logically primary concept in medicine ('disease' being derived from it rather than vice versa); and in chapter 5, the properties of 'illness', including some (though only some) of the differences between its subspecies 'mental illness' and 'physical illness', were found to be directly attributable to certain well-recognized logical properties common to all value terms.

What is required now is a more substantive account of 'illness' in its own right. It is this that will be attempted in this chapter. The line of argument, as in this section generally, will be directed towards further definition of the particular kind of value expressed by 'illness' – medical as distinct from, e.g., moral and aesthetic value. A first step towards this in respect of the closely related concept of 'dysfunction' was taken in the last chapter. Hence the argument here will start by developing a specification of 'illness' by comparing and contrasting it with the specification of 'dysfunction' developed in chapter 6. In the case of 'illness', however, this form of argument will lead not to 'function' but to 'action'. What then emerges is a kind of evolutionary theory of 'illness'. That is to say, rather than deriving a single definition, the complex and diverse properties of 'illness' in ordinary usage are shown to be understandable as developments of the concept on and from its origins in the experience of a particular kind of action failure – failure of what is here called "ordinary" doing in the apparent absence of obstruction and/or opposition. In the present chapter this account of 'illness', developed mainly from examples of physical illness, will be left to some extent schematic. But it will be developed further in chapters 8–10, in which a wide variety of examples of mental illness, together with actual case material, will be considered.

The constituents of illness, those symptoms and signs to which people refer in ascribing illness, are various. However, it is movings and not movings, as constituents of certain kinds of physical illness, which are closest to the movings and not movings of machines like cars, from which the analysis of 'dysfunction' set out in chapter 6 was mainly derived. Thus, it is by examples of illness so constituted that, in comparing and contrasting 'illness' and 'dysfunction', the similarities and differences between them will most readily be displayed. It is therefore illnesses of this kind, such as chorea, ataxia and paralysis, that we will have in mind first in this chapter. It should be emphasized, though, that this is merely a convenience. It is not intended to suggest that such illnesses are somehow logically more basic than others. On the contrary, the analysis of 'illness' obtained by considering conditions such as these, will be extended later in this chapter to other, perhaps more common and familiar, kinds of illness constituted by feelings and sensations such a pain. And the natural progression from there, feelings and sensations being mental rather than physical phenomena, will be (in chapter 8) to mental illness.

Movement and/or lack of movement as illness

As we saw in chapter 6, a car which swerves as it drives along is sometimes, but only sometimes, not functioning properly. Similarly then, a person swerving as he walks along is sometimes, but only sometimes, ill. And similar, too, up to a point, are the criteria by which are marked out, respectively, those cases of cars swerving in which they are not functioning properly and those cases of people swerving in which they are ill. Thus, in neither case will either a statistical or a reductionist specification do. This goes back to the considerations of part II. A statistical specification will not do essentially because swerving movements, although atypical, and although *sometimes* a constituent of illness, are not uniquely so. No description merely of a person's movements can mark them out as ill.

Likewise, a reductionist specification (for example, swerving is an illness if caused by some underlying bodily disease) will not do because what counts as a disease is determined by what counts as illness, not vice versa. (Note, though, that for both kinds of specification, having once *established* what counts as illness, then secondarily elaborated disease concepts – symptomatic, associative and causal – allow inferences from disease to illness, as described in chapter 4). Then again, whatever specification is proposed must cover, as much for people being ill as for cars not functioning properly, not moving (as when paralysed) as well as moving. Furthermore, at least part of what is involved in the specification of 'illness', as in the specification of 'dysfunction', is a distinction between, on the one hand, something wrong, respectively *with* persons and *with* machines, and, on the other, something (external) which is done or happens *to* them. Of course, in both cases, some more or less manifest external agency may be the cause of something wrong – and then indeed, and consistently with this part of the specification of 'illness', we speak rather of "damage" or "wounds". But as to illness a person swerving is no more ill if he has slipped or been pushed, say, than a car swerving is not functioning properly if, as in chapter 6, it has skidded or been hit by another car. Neither is a person ill if his limbs are made to jerk by an electric shock – he is not suffering from chorea. Nor is a person ill if he is merely restrained – he is not paralysed.

Here, however, the specifications of 'illness' and of 'dysfunction' diverge. To the extent that illness and dysfunction are both distinguished from things that are done or happen, to people and functional objects respectively, they are indeed similar. But illness is also distinguished *from*, where dysfunction is distinguished *as*, things that people and functional objects respectively do. A swerving person is not ill if he is, say, deliberately dodging something. Similarly, a person whose limbs are jerking (as in chorea) is not ill if he is jerking them himself. Nor is he ill when his limbs are not moving (as in paralysis) if he is either simply not moving them or actually holding them still. And here, to first appearances anyway, is something of a paradox. For a movement or a keeping-still, it would seem, should be either something that is done or happens to someone (or something) or something that the person (or thing) does. Between these alternatives there would appear to be no room for a middle term. Yet as constituents of illness, movements and keepings-still are, apparently, neither one thing nor the other.

Remember though, first, that it is only in the particular sense of 'do' in which functional objects do things in functioning (that is, 'functional do'), that dysfunctioning is distinguished as something that functional objects do (chapter 6); whereas, second, it is characteristically, though not exclusively, *people* who fall ill (chapter 2). The divergence of 'illness' from 'dysfunction' at this point thus suggests that there may be an important logical link between 'illness' and some (as yet to be defined) sense of 'do' in which people characteristically, though not exclusively, do things. Specifically, it suggests that 'illness' may stand in relation to this latter sense of 'do', much as 'dysfunction' stands in relation to 'functional do'.

The next step, in comparing and contrasting 'illness' and 'dysfunction', must therefore be to look at the senses of 'do' in which people do things. Consider first a small-scale example – I raise my arm. If I do this in the way in which people ordinarily do things, *what* I do is not specified sufficiently by a description merely of the movements of my arm. This is because although every case of my raising my arm is a case of my arm rising, not every case of my arm rising is a case of my raising my arm (for example, someone else could lift it up). In this respect the sense of 'do' in which I do something when I raise my arm, in the everyday way in which people do things, is similar to the sense of 'functional do'. And the two senses are also similar in that part at least of what else has to be specified, over and above the movements which take place, is the purpose with which what is done is done. In the case of a functional object such as a car, what has to be specified in addition to its state of motion, is its "designed-for" purpose. In the case of my raising my arm, what has to be specified, in addition to the state of motion of my arm, is my purpose in raising it. Indeed if, on raising my arm, I am asked *what* I am doing, I will probably reply not by describing myself as raising my arm but by describing my purpose in raising it. For normally (though not, for example, in the dark) the former description – that I am raising my arm – will be self-evident. Normally, therefore, it is the latter description – of my purpose in raising my arm – that is required to complete the description of what I am doing: that I am signalling a taxi, say, or making a bid or reaching for a book or stretching or exercising or merely demonstrating my raising my arm and so on.

The two kinds of 'doing' are thus similar in that both involve some idea of purpose. However, it will be clear already that the kind of purpose required to complete the specification of what a functional object does is quite different from that required to complete the specification of what I do. In the case of a functional object the purpose is that of someone or something else; it is its "designed-for" purpose, the purpose it was designed to serve. In my case, however, the required purpose is (as has already been implied) *my* purpose. Even if I am, say, signalling a taxi not for myself but for you, still *my* purpose in what *I* am doing is to signal a taxi for you. This does not mean that our purposes, yours and mine, may not coincide. Nor does it mean that in what I do I may not, sometimes without even knowing it, serve the purposes of someone or something else in addition to my own purposes. I may indeed actually function, though usually knowingly, as a doctor, say. And I may certainly be coerced. Then again, someone else may raise my arm with the purpose of serving my purposes – for example, a physiotherapist trying to restore function to my arm by means of passive arm movements. But all the same, in so far as it is *I* who do something, in so far as I am myself the agent in what I do, then it is by my purpose (together with my movings/ keepings-still) that what I do is specified.

A second difference between my raising my arm and an object functioning follows on from this. Thus the "designed-for" purpose of a functional object, however widely it is defined, is necessarily invariant: change the purpose which a functional object is designed to serve, and you change not only what it does in functioning but also what *it* is. By contrast, my purpose in what I do, even if it is something as simple as raising my arm, can vary widely; so much so, indeed, that I may, exceptionally, have no purpose at all in raising my arm. I may do it, say, simply from habit. Indeed, I regularly do certain things this way – for example, hum a tune. And this shows how different my raising my arm is not only from what a functional object does in functioning (which is by definition always purposive) but also from my arm just rising. For if I have no purpose in raising my arm, it is this – that I have no purpose in raising it – which is required to complete the specification of what I am doing. But my arm just rising, even though, contingently, it may happen that some purpose (even my purpose) is thereby served, is completely specified by 'my arm just rising'. The differences here can be thought of as being like differences between expressions in mathematics. In an expression specifying what a functional object does in functioning, its "designed-for" purpose would appear as a constant. In an expression specifying what I do in raising my arm, my purpose would appear as a variable, the possible values of which include zero (that is, having no purpose). But in an expression specifying what my arm does in just rising there would be no term for purpose at all, either constant or variable.

A third difference between the two kinds of doing also involves purpose, but indirectly. This difference consists in the fact that while there is only one sense of 'do' in which an object may do something in functioning, there are many different senses of 'do' in which I may do something in raising my arm. In some of these senses furthermore, I am, somehow, more fully or more completely doing something in raising my arm, than in others. If I raise my arm automatically (for example, swinging it up as I walk along) or instinctively (for example, to ward off a blow) or by reflex (for example, withdrawing from a painful stimulus), I am certainly doing something: but I am not doing something in as full or complete a sense as when I raise my arm, say, intentionally. Thus, although all these senses of 'do' are fully purposive, I would normally be held responsible for things that I do intentionally, but not, or not to the same degree, for things that I do automatically, instinctively, or by reflex. Furthermore, this sense of "intentional" doing, as a fuller or more complete sense of 'do' in which I may do things, goes with a fuller or more complete sense in which my purpose comes into the specification of what I do. For, if I do something intentionally, not only is the purpose which is served my purpose, but it is one of which I am, or may more or less readily become, conscious. This is so not merely in the sense that my purpose is one which may be, or may more or less readily become, known to me – as indeed my purpose in raising my arm automatically, instinctively or by reflex, may be, or may more or less readily become, known to me; but also in the sense that my purpose is one which I may have, or may more or less readily call, before my mind as, or before – sometimes long before – I act on it. And such a purpose we indeed call (though the word has other meanings as well) an intention.

' "Intentional" doing', defined in this way, is of particular interest here. For, like 'illness', it is characteristic of, but not exclusive to, people. Up to the introduction of intention, everything that had been said of me *vis-à-vis* raising my arm could have been said not only of other people but of organisms in general. Even the most lowly organisms serve their own purposes in what they do. In this, indeed, organisms in general differ from functional objects. Similarly, the purposes of even the most lowly organisms, though contingently limited, are not logically restricted (that is, by definition of what it is for an object to be an organism or an organism of a particular kind) as are the purposes of functional objects: an amoeba, say, whose purposes in doing something were as a matter of fact *not* to survive and/or reproduce (cf. chapter 3) would none the less still itself and *qua* amoeba, be doing something. But consciousness, and hence the possibility at least of doing things (in the sense here defined) intentionally, is normally attributed only to people and other organisms like people relatively high in the animal kingdom. So there is a (rough) correlation here between "intentional" doing, as a kind of doing characteristic of but not exclusive to people, and illness. Of course, there is more to the full sense of 'do' in which people may do things than just intention (as here defined). Even the very simple movement of raising one's arm may, depending on circumstances, involve voluntariness and free choice, together or separately, and in varying combinations with knowledge, foresight, self-control and so on. And most of the things people do are not as simple as this. They involve complex bodily movements and, as will be considered in detail later on, mental elements such as attention and perception (for example, listening to music). Austin, in a well-known paper (1956/7), drew attention to the variety of human action and to the relative neglect of this variety in the philosophy of action. Moreover, he pointed to abnormal psychology as an important and largely untapped resource for philosophies of action. Here, taking Austin's point the other way around, as it were, the variety of human action will emerge later on as a crucial factor determining the logical properties of 'illness'. But what matters for the moment is simply the correlation between the attribution of 'illness' and that of ' "intentional" doing'.

Now, however, it may seem that something of a retreat is called for. Thus, the conclusion that is invited by this correlation is that it is ' "intentional" doing' that stands in relation to 'illness' as ' "functional" doing' stands in relation to 'dysfunction'. But if this is so, then the original example of arm raising may appear to have been inappropriate. For if I raise my arm in, as was said, the "everyday way in which people do things", I will hardly be involved in anything so ponderous as intending to raise it, in "having or calling my purposes before my mind", let alone choosing voluntarily, acting with free will and the rest. On the contrary, if I raise my arm in the everyday way in which people do things, I will, in Austin's words, "just get on and do it". And in this respect, indeed, it may seem that the (philosophically standard) choice of a small-scale, substantially trivial example as a starting-point has been positively misleading. The reason for starting from such an example was sound enough: namely, that it is by examples of this kind that the essentially logical points with which philosophy is primarily concerned are most likely to be displayed (cf. chapter 3). But in this case, at least, if it is ' "intentional" doing' which is relevant to 'illness', then doing of this kind is normally associated with somewhat larger-scale and less substantially trivial things that people do than raising their arms. ' "Intentional" doing', along with any other full sense of 'do', is normally associated with things like being helpful to someone or writing an article or winning a prize.

However, any retreat at this stage should not be too ready or too far. In the first place, "ordinary" doing, as it will now be called, is really not so different from "intentional" doing. To say, with Austin, that in doing something one "just gets on and does it", is really to say no more than that one is not, at the time, reflecting *on* one's intentions, or indeed on any other element of the full sense of 'do'. One reflects on these elements only when one's attention is *drawn* to them. This may happen, as in the example above, if I am asked what I am doing; I may then, as was said, more or less readily call my purposes before my mind. Or it may happen when I seek to excuse something that I have done, pointing retrospectively to some respect in which my "machinery of action" (Austin's phraseology again) was somehow not fully engaged – I did not, as we say, intend to do it, or I did not do it voluntarily. The foregoing analysis of my raising my arm should thus be understood as an extension of this ordinary capacity for reflecting on, and becoming aware of, what one is doing. And it should thus be understood as showing not, as it was originally taken to be showing, that the sense of 'do' in which people ordinarily do things is the full sense of 'do', but rather as showing that this sense of 'do' is one in which the full sense is latent.

"Ordinary" doing is thus "latent full" doing. And the reason for this is clear enough – namely, that in regard to the everyday things that people do, the elements of the full sense, by which their machinery of action is comprised, operate largely trouble-free. Indeed, although one's attention may be drawn to these elements in the self-reflecting ways just described, it is most commonly and most powerfully drawn to them by difficulty. Difficulty, though, not in the task itself, for then the task itself, being inherently difficult, would *a fortiori not* be among those which one would ordinarily just get on and do. Rather, it would be something which, ordinarily, one would choose carefully to do or not to do, and which, if one chose to do it, one would do with one's purpose (to do that difficult thing) firmly before one's mind. And hence indeed the setting of one's experience of the "full" sense of 'do' mainly among the larger-scale and substantially non-trivial things that one does; these being, on the whole, the more difficult things that one does. Difficulty, then, not in the task itself, but difficulty external to it, that is to say, difficulty arising from obstruction and/or opposition. And difficulty of this external kind may arise not only in respect of things like signalling a taxi (for example, in the rain) or making a bid (for example, against competition), but even in respect of things as small-scale and substantially trivial as raising an arm. My hand may be stuck in my pocket, and raising my arm then becomes (momentarily) something that I do with my purpose (here just to raise my arm) before my mind – that is, it becomes something that I do (in this sense of the word) intentionally. Our understanding of the sense of 'do' in which people ordinarily do things is thus taken a step further. For this sense of 'do' is now seen not only to be one in which the full sense is latent, but also one in which the full sense is made overt – most commonly and most powerfully made overt – by obstruction and/or opposition.

This brings the argument back to 'illness'. Thus, to the extent that ' "ordinary" doing' is a sense of 'do' in which the elements of the full sense are latent, the attribution of ' "ordinary" doing' follows that of ' "intentional" doing' in being correlated with the attribution of 'illness'. To this extent, then, ' "ordinary" doing' is as good a candidate as ' "intentional" doing' to stand in relation to 'illness' as ' "functional" doing' stands in relation to 'dysfunction'. When it comes to *failure* of doing, however, ' "ordinary" doing', as a sense of 'do' in which the elements of the full sense are made overt by obstruction and/or opposition, has a distinct edge. For a failure to do something which is inherently difficult will normally be experienced as just that – as a failure, usually in some full sense of 'do', to do that difficult thing. But a failure to do something which is *not* inherently difficult, a failure to do something which one would ordinarily just get on and do, will normally be experienced as something one has been prevented from doing by obstruction and/or opposition. Hence, "obstruction and/or opposition" comes out on both sides of the experiential fence. In the face of obstruction and/or opposition, *successfully* doing something which one would ordinarily just get on and do, is normally experienced as really *doing* something, i.e., as doing something in the full sense of 'do'; whereas *failing* in these circumstances is normally experienced as being *prevented* from doing it. But this latter experience translates into the terminology used earlier in respect of 'illness', as the experience of something being done (opposition) or happening (obstruction) *to* one. I go to raise my arm, and someone, say, tries to stop me: then either I succeed in raising it, in which case I really do (in the full sense) *do* something; or I fail, in which case something is done *to* me. Hence, the experiences of "doing" and of "done/happens to" will tend, in respect of the things one ordinarily just gets on and does, to become contrasted. And consider, therefore, the experience of failing to do something which one would ordinarily just get on and do, but in the *absence* of obstruction and/or opposition. This, like the experience of illness, will be a somewhat paradoxical experience. For, like illness, it will be experienced neither as something that one *does* nor as something that is done or happens *to* one.

The retreat, therefore, of a few pages back, is now seen to have been no more than a tactical retreat, leading as it has not only to a clearer understanding of the sense of 'do' in which people ordinarily do things, but also, and by the same token, to a closer approach to the target concept of 'illness'. For ' "ordinary" doing' is now seen to be correlated with 'illness' not only in its attribution, but also in respect of the properties of the experience of failure. To draw a correlation, of course, even to draw two, is not to make a connection. However, the correlations drawn here have at least a good logical pedigree. For they have come out not coincidentally but in a direct line of descent from the strategy adopted at the start of the chapter – namely, of analysing 'illness' by comparing and contrasting it with 'dysfunction'. Furthermore, the main steps, from strategy to correlations, have followed one another quite naturally. First came the recognition that 'illness', although similar to 'dysfunction' in being distinguished from things that are done or happen respectively to people and to functional objects, none the less differs from it in being also distinguished from, where 'dysfunction' is distinguished as, something that people and functional objects respectively do. Then came the recollection, from chapter 6, that it is only in that particular sense of 'do' in which functional objects do things (' "functional" doing' as it was called) that 'dysfunction' is distinguished as something that functional objects do. From this came the consideration of the senses of 'do' in which people do things, since it is people rather than functional objects who fall ill. And from this came the correlations.

The connection between 'illness' and ' "ordinary" doing' which is suggested by these correlations is, however, like the connection found in chapter 6 between 'dysfunction' and ' "functional" doing', a logical connection, a connection of meaning. Hence, combining this with the conclusion of chapter 4, that among medical concepts it is 'illness' rather than 'disease' or 'dysfunction' which is logically primary, shows that the kind of connection which is suggested by these correlations is not merely a logical connection but a logically primary connection. It is a connection, that is to say, at the very origins of the medical concepts, one from which these concepts, by way originally of 'illness', are actually derived. That there should be a connection of this logically primitive or original kind between 'illness' and ' "ordinary" doing' is, in relation to 'illness' at least (as distinct from 'disease'), not at all far-fetched. Flew (1973, Part II), in particular, has emphasized the logical priority in medicine of the notion of incapacity. And is not the first intimation of illness often just this – that of finding oneself unable, although not obstructed and/or opposed, to do things which one would ordinarily just get on and do? So here, at least, the first intimation of illness is indeed no less than the experience of failure of "ordinary" doing in the absence of obstruction and/or opposition. And as to finding oneself unable in the absence of obstruction and/or opposition, to do even so ordinary a thing as raise one's arm, well, one's first recourse would surely be to go straight to one's doctor!

Mark you, once in the doctor's surgery, the lessons of chapter 4 would have to be borne in mind if the connection between 'illness' and ' "ordinary" doing' is to remain visible. For as we saw in chapter 4, one's doctor is likely to be concerned primarily (and properly) not (or not directly) with whether one is ill but with what disease one might be suffering from. He is likely to be concerned, that is, with "disease diagnosis", not with "illness diagnosis"; with the identification of one's inability to raise one's arm with one or more of those particular conditions widely regarded as illnesses (defined partly symptomatically, partly by associated signs, and partly causally) with which doctors are currently familiar. For it is in this way that one's doctor is most likely to be able effectively to tackle the immediate empirical problem of what to do about one's inability to raise one's arm. But these concerns, with disease, are, according to the argument of chapter 4, logically derivative on a concern with illness. And this remains true, even though, as described in chapter 4, the disease concepts, once derived, can operate often with a degree of apparent independence (as in speaking of someone having a disease even though he is not, at the time, ill; cf. p. 65). So that, all in all, while it is 'disease', not 'illness', which for the best of practical reasons is uppermost in the doctor's mind, and while the doctor, in making a diagnosis, will therefore not usually be thinking in terms of "ordinary" (or any other kind of) doing, this is in no way prejudicial to the suggestion that there may be some logically primary link between ' "ordinary" doing' and 'illness'. On the contrary, the suggestion is rather strongly, if indirectly, supported by this observation. For even in chapter 1 it was anticipated that the concept of 'illness' was likely to be found hidden beneath a veil of the more familiar concepts of 'disease', that it might well appear unfamiliar when we got to it, and that getting to it would require no small effort of imagination.

But there is also a good deal of more direct support, of this first outcome criterion kind, for the existence of a logically primary link between 'illness' and ' "ordinary" doing'. In the first place, if the logical origins of the medical concepts are indeed in the experience of failure of ' "ordinary" doing', then a number of features of the ordinary use of these concepts which had to be left unexplained at the end of chapter 5, can now be seen to be no more than results of the natural development of these concepts on and from their origins. After all, concepts generally are not, as it were, evolutionarily static. They bud and branch and interconnect, forming what Witt-

genstein described as families of concepts linked by a complicated network of similarities overlapping and criss-crossing
(1958, paras. 65–7). One such family of concepts we have
traced already – namely, the whole complex of disease concepts described in chapter 4, developed under selective pressures arising from the empirical demands of clinical practice.
Another, rather differently-based, development is that by
which medical concepts have come to be used of plants and
animals. The development of disease concepts in medicine
(according to the argument of chapter 4) was mainly by way of
linking (statistically, causally and so on) conditions widely
regarded as illnesses (that is, conditions in the subcategory Id) to
other conditions. The use of medical concepts in respect of
plants and animals, on the other hand, can be understood as
having developed more straightforwardly by way of Wittgensteinian-style cross-similarities (symptomatic similarities, causal
similarities and so on) between them and people. There is of
course no logically hard-and-fast or final process at work here.
In principle any similarity might do; and which similarities or
groups of similarities have so far actually been involved, is as
much a matter of psychology as of logic. Furthermore, the
process is not all or nothing. There is often, therefore, especially
with very lowly organisms, a distinct element of "as if" in our
use of the medical concepts in respect of them: is a bacterium
invaded by a phage really diseased, for example? Or is it
wounded or infested or simply damaged or what? None the
less, it is in terms of cross-similarities that we are able to
understand why a plant eaten by a leaf-mould, say, is said to
have a disease, while one which is eaten by a caterpillar or a
cow is simply said to be eaten.

It is, however, more particularly in the constraints on the
development of the medical concepts, rather than in their
development as such, that signs of their logical origins specifically in ' "ordinary" doing' are most readily discernible. Here,
too, plants and animals provide a case in point. For one such
constraint is the restriction (first noted in chapter 2) of the use
of 'illness' mainly to higher animals, especially "pets", notwithstanding the use of 'disease' more or less indifferently of plants
and animals in general. One reason for this restriction, that

noted in chapter 4, is that it is mainly only of higher animals, especially of "pets", that we have things to say which are served better by the more evaluative connotations of 'illness' than the more factual connotations of 'disease'. But in tracing the logical origin of the medical concepts – by way, remember, of 'illness' – to the experience of failure of ' "ordinary" doing', we have a second, more powerful reason. For "ordinary" doing – and hence the experience of failure of "ordinary" doing – is attributed mainly only to people and to animals like people relatively high in the animal kingdom. Thus, if the use of the medical concepts in respect of plants and animals is dependent on Wittgensteinian-style cross-similarities between them and people, then, while there will often be sufficient (symptomatic, causal and so on) cross-similarities for the logically derivative disease concepts to be used of plants and animals in general, in the case of 'illness' the similarities will be sufficient only for organisms like people relatively high in the animal kingdom, i.e., for higher animals; and if this is especially so for "pets", clearly because of our identification with them, as was said in chapter 4, in some respects actually as people. Hence, even if, contrary to the general rule relied on in chapter 4, we have things to say of lower organisms which might otherwise have been well served by the more evaluative connotations of 'illness', our use of 'illness' in respect of such organisms will tend to be inhibited by Wittgensteinian-style cross-*dis*similarities between them and people. And indeed, where 'illness' is so used (though more often it is some less specific term like 'sick' or 'ailing' that is employed), the element of "as if" is normally so prominent as to render the meaning of what is said definitely metaphorical.

Somewhat similar constraints, arising from Wittgensteinian-style cross-dissimilarities, are to be found in our ordinary use of the medical concepts in respect of functional objects, biological and non-biological. Functional objects, indeed, together with organisms like plants and animals, form here something of a progression: from organisms themselves, in respect of (at least) the higher varieties of which we use both 'illness' and 'disease', through biological functional objects (like lungs, legs, livers and so on) in respect of which (other than metaphorically) we use only 'disease'; to non-biological functional objects such as machines, in respect of which (other than metaphorically) we use neither 'illness' nor 'disease'. And this progression, as can now be seen, corresponds with a progression in logical distance, as it were, from the (here proposed) origins of the medical concepts in the experience of failure of ' "ordinary" doing'. Thus lower organisms, by virtue of mainly quantitative differences (for example, in the attribution of conscious purposes), are further than higher organisms from these origins; but functional objects, by virtue of at least one further, and qualitative, difference (namely, that their purposes, unlike those of organisms, are not their own), are further still; and whereas in the case of biological functional objects (which anyway are parts of organisms) this qualitative difference has been partly bridged by connections of the (statistical or causal) kind outlined in chapter 4, in the case of non-biological functional objects it has not been. Or at any rate not yet. For the development of the medical concepts, as has been emphasized, is not subject to hard-and-fast or final processes. And indeed, as non-biological functional objects become more organism-like, as machines become more person-like, we may expect to see the "as if" element in our use of the medical concepts in respect of them recede, perhaps eventually disappearing altogether. But given the progression just outlined, the fact that this has not happened so far is at least consistent with the suggestion that the logical origins of the medical concepts are in the experience of failure of "ordinary" doing.

Yet a third kind of constraint, also consistent with these origins, is illustrated by the conditions mentioned in chapter 6: death, disability, old age and being just unfit. For each of these conditions, although a dysfunctional condition, and a dysfunctional condition not least of higher organisms including people, is nevertheless logically distinct not only from illness but also from disease. And part at least of what is involved here can now be traced to the (proposed) logical origins of the medical concepts in the experience of failure of "ordinary" doing, or, more specifically, to the expectations of just getting on and doing things, upon which ' "ordinary" doing', and hence the experience of failure of "ordinary" doing, depend. These

expectations, consistently with its here proposed logical priority, are transparently present in our use of 'illness', at least of
the moving/not moving kind considered so far. Thus, it is only
because of the *expectation* that (in the absence of obstruction
and/or opposition) one will just get on and raise one's arm, that
failure to do so will lead one straight to the doctor. Similarly, it
is by reference to such expectations, such experientially derived
individual expectations, that, as we saw more fully in chapter 3,
illness can be said to involve a departure from "the norm".
Indeed, in connecting 'illness' (logically) with the experience of
failure of "ordinary" doing, the present analysis automatically
follows ordinary use in excluding as symptoms of illness
failures to do things which one would *not* ordinarily expect to
do – not merely things like running up three flights of stairs
without shortness of breath when one has not been taking
regular exercise and is thus "just unfit", or is very old or very
young; but also, whether young and fit or not, things like
running a mile in four minutes, let alone (as we are presently
constituted) flying unaided or seeing in the ultraviolet. But
aside from 'illness', even in our use of the logically derivative
'disease' there are echoes or residues of these expectations. One
example of this is the distinction between disease and disability.
Thus, so long as there is at least some expectation of change
(whether for better or worse, spontaneous or iatrogenic),
someone with even a very chronically disabling condition, such
as multiple sclerosis, will be thought of as having a disease;
whereas with an essentially static condition such as that which
may follow poliomyelitis, and with a condition which therefore results in a permanent change in one's expectations of what
one can "just get on and do", they will be thought of simply as
being disabled. While as to death, in a sense the ultimate
disability, this, of course, is finally permanent.

At this point, though, it may once again be thought that the
argument is at risk of overreaching itself and that a second
retreat is therefore called for. For now, in coming on to talk of
conditions of this last "dysfunctional" kind, it will be realized
that the condition from which the argument of the last few
paragraphs sprang – the condition of finding oneself unable to
raise one's arm – is itself as likely to be regarded as a

dysfunctional condition as an illness. After all, it could be pointed out, is not my complaint with such a condition as likely to be that there is something wrong with my arm – that it is not "functioning" properly – as it is to be that I am ill? And with such a condition, therefore, is there not, in the present analysis, a risk of falling between two stools? Between, on the one hand, smaller-scale conditions less equivocally thought of as dysfunctional conditions – conditions such as some particular muscle group failing to contract properly or, smaller-scale still, nerve-to-muscle chemical messenger substances failing to be released properly at the nerve-muscle junction – and, on the other hand, larger-scale conditions, not so well circumscribed and more whole-body conditions, less equivocally thought of as illnesses; conditions, indeed, like that mentioned right at the start of this chapter, of finding oneself (unaccountably) swerving as one walks along? Of course, the consideration, here, of the equivocal "failure of arm raising" is a result, merely, of the original philosophically standard choice of arm raising as an example from which to launch into the philosophy of action. But now, with hindsight, it may be said, would our purpose not have been better served by some other, larger-scale example?

This second retreat however, is, as the first turned out to be, only a tactical retreat. For it leads directly back to one of two main questions left outstanding at the end of chapter 5 – namely, how the relationship between 'dysfunction' and 'illness' should be understood. The key to this is that just as failure of arm raising is equivocal as to 'dysfunction' and 'illness', so arm raising itself is equivocal as to ' "functional" doing' and to ' "ordinary" doing'. Failure to move my arm may be construed either as something wrong with me – I am ill – or as something wrong with my arm – my arm is not functioning properly. Similarly, movement of my arm may be construed either as me "ordinarily" doing something – I move my arm – or as my arm "functionally" doing something – my arm moves. And from this matching of equivocations it follows that if 'illness' is indeed derived from ' "ordinary" doing' in the way suggested in this chapter and 'dysfunction' from ' "functional" doing' in the way suggested in chapter 6, then the

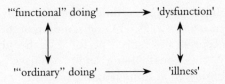

The relationship between 'illness' and 'dysfunction'
If 'dysfunction' is derived (logically) from ' "functional" doing' and
'illness' from ' "ordinary" doing', then the equivocation between
'illness' and 'dysfunction' in ordinary usage corresponds with (and
is to be understood in terms of) that between ' "functional" doing'
and ' "ordinary" doing'.

relationship between 'illness' and 'dysfunction' is to be understood in terms of the relationship between ' "ordinary" doing'
and ' "functional" doing'. And this, indeed, amounts to further
first outcome-criterion support for the existence of a logical
link between 'illness' and ' "ordinary" doing'. For, if ' "ordinary" doing' and ' "functional" doing' are equivocal this way,
then the equivocal relationship of 'illness' and 'dysfunction', as
a feature of the ordinary use of the medical concepts, drops
irresistibly out of a theory placing ' "ordinary" doing' in much
the same relationship to 'illness' as ' "functional" doing' stands
in relationship to 'dysfunction'.

From one point of view, to say this may be thought to say
rather little. For what it amounts to is only to push the question
back a step, from the question of how one relationship (that
between 'dysfunction' and 'illness') should be understood, to
the question of how another relationship (that between
' "functional" doing' and ' "ordinary" doing') should be
understood. And the latter relationship could hardly be
thought to be any less obscure and intractable than the former!
Furthermore, if the latter relationship is obscure and intractable, it is clear that any full consideration of it will involve
some consideration of the yet more obscure and intractable
relationship between persons and their bodies; for it is "*I* do"
which is set up against "my arm does", and it is *I* who fall ill,
but my arm which fails to function properly (see also chapter
11). From another point of view, though, to say this, at this
now quite far advanced stage of the argument, is to say a lot.

For, constrained as the argument has been by our main objective – to achieve a clearer understanding of the specifically medical concepts – and indeed perforce of this objective, the concepts of ' "functional" doing' and ' "ordinary" doing' have had to be considered at some length. And if the pictures so far plotted of these two concepts have been essentially separate pictures, still, sufficient detail has already been filled in to show at least one possible route by which the relationship between them might be explored.

This is an important growth point for the argument, and to follow its implications right through would involve a large study in its own right. However, the main steps might be these. The argument could start from the concept of 'purpose', as an element common to both pictures, and, in both, serving the same end – namely, that of marking out the two kinds of doing ("functional" doing and "ordinary" doing) from other effects respectively of functional objects and people or other organisms (remember the "adventitious properties" of functional objects in chapter 6 and "my purpose" in this chapter). Next, the various examples of the two kinds of doing accumulated in this chapter could be lined up together, side by side. This would show that the purposes by which these examples are severally defined are connected by (perceived) cause–effect links: I signal a taxi, *by* raising my arm, *by* my arm muscles contracting, *by* chemical-messenger substances being released from the nerve-muscle junctions in my arm and so on. The analysis proper could then begin with an examination of these links, as links in the relationship between ' "ordinary" doing' and ' "functional" doing'. This analysis would seek *inter alia* to explain (what is no doubt a matter as much of psychology as of logic) how it is that on any particular occasion of my raising my arm, even though each of the links in the chain is in *some* sense something that I am doing, one or more of them is picked out to be, as it was put, my more or less conscious purpose; and hence to be the particular purpose by which (on that occasion) what I am ("ordinarily") doing is defined; and then to explain why it should be that the more proximal of these links, those further up the chain, are more likely to be so picked out than those that are more distal (it requires very special circumstances, a neurophysiological experiment perhaps, for my more or less conscious purpose in raising my arm to be to release chemical neurotransmitter substances; and circumstances such as these, incidentally, raise nice questions about the direction of the cause–effect links in the chain itself); and from this to explain how it is that, in this respect, purposes like arm raising are intermediate in position, being neither distal nor proximal, and, hence, equivocal; and so to explain generally how *my* purpose is related to the purpose of my arm (which relation, as is shown not least by equivocal cases of this kind, is not or not simply that of cause and effect); and thus to explain (something of) how I am related to my body; and, so on . . . : and in all this, or in any part of it (for it amounts to a tall order, certainly), to be exploring not merely the relationship between ' "ordinary" doing' and ' "functional" doing', but, by implicit extension, that between 'illness' and 'dysfunction' as well.

Pushing the question back a step, therefore, from that of the relationship between 'illness' and 'dysfunction' to that of the relationship between ' "ordinary" doing' and ' "functional" doing', is very far from being heuristically empty. For although this manoeuvre raises as many difficulties as it solves, these difficulties are inherent in the former relationship just as much as in the latter; and as difficulties in the latter relationship they are susceptible if not of solution, at least of further investigation by way of studies of the cause–effect chain of purposes connecting ' "functional" doing' with ' "ordinary" doing'. This, then, gives an approach to one of the two main questions left still outstanding at the end of chapter 5. And if the chain of purposes is now traced the other way, forwards *from* ' "ordinary" doing', rather than back to ' "functional" doing', an approach to the other main question becomes apparent, the question indeed which is the target question in this chapter, namely how the particular kind of value which is expressed by the medical concepts should be characterized.

There are four main steps along the route to this second question. Step 1 is to notice the tendency as the chain of purposes is traced forwards, for the evaluative element in its meaning to become more and more overt. This tendency has to some extent been anticipated by certain differences implicit in the things said respectively about ' "functional" doing' in chapter 6 and ' "ordinary" doing' in this chapter. In chapter 6 in particular, a long argument was required in order to expose the evaluative element in the meaning of ' "functional" doing' as applied to non-biological functional objects. This element was eventually located at one remove from the objects themselves, in the intentions of their designers. In this chapter, on the other hand, the corresponding evaluative element in the meaning of ' "ordinary" doing', as applied mainly to people, has been found to be much nearer the surface of the concept, in the more or less conscious purposes with which people themselves ("ordinar-ily") do things. Furthermore, this difference between ' "func-tional" doing' and ' "ordinary" doing' corresponds with the fact that 'illness' itself is a more overtly evaluative concept than 'dysfunction' (this was the basis of Boorse's analysis, it will be recalled). And if the argument of this chapter linking 'illness' with ' "ordinary" doing' is right, it is also one which helps to explain this fact.

But to return to step 1. If the chain of purposes is now traced forwards from ' "ordinary" doing', what is found is that the evaluative element in its meaning comes not just up to the surface but right out into the open. For what is found is that the expressions by which successive purposes are defined become increasingly likely actually to be evaluative expressions: why signal a taxi? – to be *helpful* to someone; why make a bid? – to get something of *value* to me. And after that the very links in the chain itself cease to be purposes and intentions as such, and become precepts, moral and otherwise, and preferences, aes-thetic and otherwise: why be helpful to someone? – because it is the *right* thing to do; why is that for which I make a bid of value to me? – because it is *beautiful*. And from this it follows (as step 2) that it is from precepts and preferences of this kind that the evaluative element in the meaning of the whole chain is (ultimately) derived, each purpose in the (cause–effect) chain being of instrumental value as a (perceived) means to the (moral or aesthetic) ends defined by the precepts and prefer-ences to which the chain itself leads. Hence (step 3), the kind of value which is implicit in the meaning of ' "ordinary" doing', being drawn as it is from a purpose or purposes in a chain of this kind, is itself instrumental value. And hence (step 4), if 'illness' is indeed derived from ' "ordinary" doing', then, to the extent that instrumental value is distinct from moral and aesthetic value, so also (and consistently with ordinary usage) will moral and aesthetic value be distinct from the kind of value which is expressed by 'illness'.

By means of these steps, then, our second question has now been set up like the first, in a form in which it is at least susceptible to further investigation. In this instance, however, rather more progress has been made towards answering it. For the proposed derivation of 'illness' from ' "ordinary" doing', explains in principle not only the fact that the kind of value which is expressed by 'illness' is distinct from moral and aesthetic value, but also certain other of its properties. Thus, in being derived from *failure* of ' "ordinary" doing', the kind of value expressed by 'illness' is necessarily negative value. Similarly, in being derived from failure of ' "*ordinary*" doing', illness itself is necessarily attributed (as ' "ordinary" doing' is atttributed) to living as opposed to non-living things, and, as noted earlier in this chapter, typically though not exclusively to people. It is worth adding that the derivation of 'illness' from 'action' also explains a further property of 'illness' – namely, its property of serving as an excuse, moral and/or legal. But for that see chapter 10.

There is more to be said about all this, of course. But from this point onwards the further investigation of the particular kind of value which is expressed by 'illness' raises, rather as the first question raised, difficulties of a general philosophical nature. In this instance, the difficulties are more in the area of moral philosophy than in that of the philosophy of action. The traditional moral philosophical problem of the freedom of the will, for example, comes in here in a particularly acute form. Any full account of the particular kind of value which is expressed by 'illness' must (in principle) address the question of how it is that this (assumed) freedom, implicit in ' "ordinary" doing' and overt in the full sense of 'doing', arises; and thus how it comes to be denied in the failure of ' "ordinary" doing' from which 'illness' (it is suggested here) is derived. For this freedom seems here to be built into our conceptual scheme with an intimate logical connection of some kind to a cause–effect chain (of purpose) which is, in a sense, its deterministic antithesis. How, then, do these two ideas (illusions?) coexist? Is the evaluative element in the meaning of the chain important in this respect? If so, how? It is by this element, as has been seen, that links in the chain are marked out not merely as causes and effects but *as* purposes. And presumably the logical independence of description and evaluation (discussed in chapter 3) may be relevant in some way to the sense (whatever this is) in which to act on purpose may be to act freely. But if so, how is this freedom related to the apparently more mechanistic nature of (the also purposive) ' "functional" doing'? Intractable difficulties indeed, then. And so there is at least cold comfort to be taken from the fact that it is the intractability of such difficulties which lies behind the more parochial medical problem of further characterizing the particular kind of value which is expressed by 'illness'.

We have now come a long way. Before going on, therefore, it may be helpful to review the course that has been followed after comparing and contrasting 'illness' and 'dysfunction' at the start of this chapter. First, an examination of the sense of 'do' in which people may do things – everyday things like raising their arms – led to the recognition of a correlation between the attribution of illness and the attribution of the full sense of 'do' in which people may do things. A first retreat, which turned out really to be just a more careful look at the example of arm raising, then led to two further correlations: the first between the ascription of 'illness' and that of the "ordinary" (or "latent full") sense of 'do' in which people may do things; the second between the properties of 'illness' and those of ' "ordinary" doing', or rather of the experience of failure of "ordinary" doing in the absence of obstruction and/ or opposition. From these correlations came the idea that there might be a logically important link between 'illness' and ' "ordinary" doing', specifically, that the logical origin of 'illness' might be in the experience of failure of "ordinary" doing in the (perceived) absence of obstruction and/or opposition. And with this came explanations for a whole series of previously unexplained features of the ordinary use not only of 'illness' but also of its derivative, 'disease'. Now, finally, with a second retreat, with a second more careful look back at the example of arm raising, ' "ordinary" doing' has come to be seen not in isolation but in context – that is, the context supplied by the purpose(s) by which it is defined being embedded in a cause–effect chain of purposes. Tracing this chain back to ' "functional" doing' has provided an approach to the first of the two questions still outstanding at the end of chapter 5, namely how the relationship between 'illness' and 'dysfunction' should be understood; while tracing it forwards to the precepts and preferences to which it leads has provided an approach to the second question, the target question in this chapter, how the particular kind of value which is expressed by 'illness' should be characterized.

Sensation and/or lack of sensation as illness

Thus far we have been concerned only with that rather restricted class of illnesses constituted by movement and/or lack of movement. That illnesses of this kind should have been considered first was dictated by our initial strategy in this chapter of comparing and contrasting 'illness' with 'dysfunction', since, as was said, it is illnesses of this kind that are closest to the dysfunctional conditions (of machines) considered in chapter 6. But, as was indeed noted, the more common and familiar kinds of illness are those constituted by feelings and sensations such as pain. Furthermore, it will be apparent that movings and not movings, as things people do, are, as constituents of illness, perhaps particularly well suited to the present analysis, i.e., to an analysis which traces the logical origins of 'illness' to "ordinary" (or indeed to any other kind) of doing. Certain other constituents of illness, it is true, are *prima facie* assimilable to such an analysis. Perceivings and not perceivings, for example, are in a sense things that people do. We say, "I see . . . "; we tell people to "look for it" and to "listen carefully"; and we speak similarly of touch, taste and smell. Perceivings and not perceivings, therefore, are in such respects conceptually similar to movings and not movings. But feelings and sensations, at least of the kinds (like pain) by which illnesses are commonly constituted, are not like this at all. They are not things that people do. We do not say "I pain", but "I am in pain"; not "I hurt", but "my leg or tooth hurts". Hence, where perceivings and not perceivings as constituents of illness are *prima facie* assimilable to the present analysis, it might seem that feelings and sensations (and their respective negatives) are not.

Now, it should be said straightaway that there is no philosophical necessity for illness constituted by feelings and sensations to be assimilable to an analysis of 'illness' derived from illnesses quite differently constituted. Indeed, as previously noted, Wittgenstein would have warned against presupposing that any such assimilation is possible, let alone necessary. For, he would have said, one should not expect to find any single or unique concept standing behind so rich a diversity of ordinary usage as is presented by the medical concepts. On the contrary, one's expectation should be of a network of concepts "overlapping and criss-crossing". Such a network, of course, has in fact already been defined. And indeed, in some circumstances at least, the attachment of feelings and sensations to the medical concepts may be understood straightforwardly in terms of one or other part of this network. To say "I feel ill", for example, may be to say no more than that I am experiencing feelings which I know to be associated (statistically associated, rather as in HDf3, in chapter 4) with diseased conditions – sometimes with a specific diseased condition – of my body. Hence, to say "I feel ill" may be to say no more than "*perhaps* I am ill", meaning "perhaps I have one or other of these diseases". Then again, to say "I feel ill" after, say, eating too much, may be to say no more than that I am experiencing feelings which are *like* those which I experience when I am ill (but without actually implying that, then and there, I am, or even may be, ill). Or 'I feel ill' may be used to mean just that I feel ghastly, this being how I usually feel when I feel ill. In ordinary usage, moreover, any or all of these meanings may be combined. And any or all of them, alone or in combination, can slip from being expressed by 'I feel ill' to being expressed by 'I am ill.'

All the same, there really are illnesses constituted by feelings and sensations, and, *prima facie*, in much the same way as there are illnesses constituted by movement. Thus, migraine and neuralgia are constituted by pain in much the same way as chorea and ataxia are constituted by movement. The situation is obscured rather more in the case of feelings and sensations by the fact that, in respect of these, disease-theory is dominant, at least in medical usage. So much is known about the bodily changes underlying feelings and sensations as illnesses, that doctors are mainly concerned with the diseases defined in terms of these changes, rather than with the feelings and sensations as such. The same is true to some extent of movement as illness, of course, but less so. To the patient, however, whose dominant concept remains 'illness', it is clear that the experience of illness may be constituted by a wide range of feelings and sensations – besides pain, there is itching, dizziness, paraesthesiae (tingling), breathlessness, tiredness and so forth. Moreover, corresponding with lack of movement, as in paralysis, lack of feelings and sensations may be constitutive of illness, as in certain kinds of degenerative nerve disorders. Notwithstanding the Wittgensteinian caveat, therefore, the *prima-facie* correspondence in ordinary medical usage of movement with all this variety of feelings and sensations places the onus firmly on philosophical theory to explain either how all these are related as species of illness or how they have come to appear to be related.

In the theory presented here, it turns out that they are related. The essential point from which this arises is that although feelings and sensations are not things that we *do*, they are things we do something *about* – withdrawing from pain, scratching an itch, steadying ourselves when we feel dizzy, changing position with paraesthesiae, catching our breath with breathlessness, going to sleep when tired and so on. Hence, feelings and sensations are built into the structure of our actions, albeit differently from movements. Though in this respect, indeed, they are really rather like movement conceptually. For movement, too, so far as "ordinary" or any other species of purposive doing is concerned, is not (simply) something we do. *Non*-purposive movement, such as a stone rolling down a hillside, is something the stone (simply) does. But for a movement to be something we (in the sense of ' "ordinary" doing') do, it too has to be built into the structure of our actions. This is the burden of much of this chapter and the last, that there is more to purposive movement (such as cars moving or people moving their arms) than the movement alone: there is purpose, and, in the case of people at least, there is more even than purpose; as noted previously there is consciousness, voluntariness, self-control, knowledge, foresight and so on, all the elements, indeed, of Austin's "machinery of action".

In relation to ' "ordinary" doing', therefore, which in the present theory is the kind of doing from which 'illness' is derived, movement and feelings and sensations are alike in being built into the structure of our actions. There is thus in the present theory at least the possibility – there is the conceptual wherewithal – for 'illness' constituted by feelings and sensations to be derived from the experience of failure of "ordinary" doing in the absence of obstruction and/or opposition ("action failure", for short), much as, according to the argument presented here, 'illness' constituted by movement is so derived. There are differences between the two kinds of illness constituent, of course. Movement, for example, is executive; it is that, *inter alia* (see next chapter), *by* which we do things. But this is all par for the course. For if there are differences in the ways in which movements on the one hand, and feelings and sensations on the other, are built into the structure of our actions, this provides in principle for there to be differences – conceptual differences, of course – in the kinds of illnesses which are derived from the two kinds of "action failure". The broad picture that emerges, then, is not of an assimilation of illness constituted by feelings and sensations to illness constituted by movement, but rather of the two kinds of illness being equal subspecies of a general concept defined in terms of "action failure". The similarities between them are then explicable in terms of their common origin in "action failure", while the differences come from differences in the ways in which their respective illness constituents are built into the structure of our actions in the first place.

This is intended merely as a sketch of how the argument of the preceding subsection might be extended to feelings and sensations. But the sketch can be filled out a little by considering rather more comprehensively how pain as a constituent of illness is marked off from pain generally. This question is equivalent to the question about movement posed at the start of this chapter; for just as not all movements are constituents of illness, neither are all pains. To answer the question, however, involves going back over much of the ground covered both in this section and in the last. And this is only what is to be expected if 'pain-as-illness' is indeed a conceptual species of the same general type as 'movement-as-illness'. Thus, one might ask first whether a factual criterion would do. And this, following the arguments of chapter 2, would lead to the conclusion that at least such factual criteria as are thrown up by conventional theories of the meaning of 'illness' – descriptive, causal and so on – will not do. Then, rather than searching for some other more subtle factual criterion, an argument of the kind outlined in chapter 3 could be employed leading to the hypothesis, introduced at the start of chapter 4, that the required criterion is not factual at all, but evaluative. For, it could be pointed out, pain, although very widely negatively evaluated, is not necessarily so evaluated; which means that there is at least the possibility that pain-as-illness is marked out as negatively evaluated pain. And from this hypothesis all the results of chapters 4 and 5 would follow, not the least of which – and which in respect of pain is that much more transparent – would be the logical priority of 'illness' over 'disease'.

Yet it would be clear from the start, as it was clear at the start of chapter 4, that such a criterion is at best over-comprehensive. For not all negatively evaluated pain is illness. And to the extent that pain-as-illness is marked out as negatively evaluated pain, the evaluation in question is not, as was noted at the end of chapter 5, negative moral or aesthetic value. So that in suggesting an evaluative criterion for pain-as-illness, it would be necessary to develop the criterion further, much as it has been developed in this chapter and the last, by exploring the particular kind of value which is expressed by 'illness'.

This further exploration could then be carried out, essentially, by way of an argument which, granted that pain is unlike movement in being something one does something *about*, would otherwise parallel the argument developed in this chapter for movement-as-illness. What one does about pain, it would be said, is to withdraw. And pain-as-illness then becomes pain from which one is unable to withdraw, not – as when one's hand is held in the flame – because of something that is done or happens to one; not – as when one holds one's own hand in a flame – because of something one does (or, here, fails to do); but (as with migraine and neuralgia) in the absence of either of these. Pain-as-illness, that is to say, is pain from which one is unable to withdraw in the (perceived) absence of obstruction and/or opposition. Of course, one difference between the argument in respect of pain as a constituent of illness and that in respect of movement is in the kind of 'doing' involved. Withdrawal from pain is well towards the reflex end of the scale of kinds of 'doing'. However, its connection with "ordinary" doing is clear from the fact that, where obstructed or opposed, withdrawal from pain becomes very clearly something one does in the full sense of 'do' – that is, with one's purpose before one's mind and so on. And from this flow all the further results of the analysis of movement-as-illness: the same somewhat paradoxical properties of 'illness'; the same experientially derived personal norms (one important condition for a pain, or any other sensation, to be experienced as a symptom of illness is normally that it be "out of the ordinary" as to quality, strength or duration); and the same differential distributions (for example, as to the use of 'illness' of plants, animals and machines). Furthermore, there is a similar equivocation: thus, when I touch something hot, "I have hurt my hand", or, "my hand hurts me". Moreover, this equivocation, as in the case of movement, reflects a chain of purposes from biological functions to conscious intentions. In the case of pain, the relevant purpose is restricted, which is another conceptual difference. But the same scope exists for exploring in terms of this chain, both the relationship between 'illness' and 'dysfunction' and the nature of the particular kind of value expressed by 'illness'; the latter coming out as before, as (negative) instrumental value derived from 'action failure' as here defined.

Let it be said again that there is no philosophical necessity for the two kinds of illness concept, 'movement-as-illness' and 'feelings/sensations-as-illness', to be assimilable in this way to a common concept of 'illness'. It is consistent with ordinary usage that they should be so; indeed, ordinary usage is explained by their being so. But that they should be so is not pre-ordained. Again, there is clearly more to be said, not only about pain as a constituent of illness but also about other feelings and sensations as constituents of illness, to fill out the sketch of the argument given here. The sketch, however, with mental illness in mind, is sufficient. For what it amounts to, as we will see more clearly in the next chapter, is a mini-generalization of the kind required for the larger generalization from 'physical illness' to 'mental illness'. Rather than spend more time on 'physical illness', therefore, we will now turn to 'mental illness'. Though the argument, not only of the next chapter but also of chapters 9 and 10, will serve to fill out the sketch presented here, by examining the wide range of mental phenomena by which the diverse species of 'mental illness' are constituted.

The reverse-view analysis of the medical concepts developed so far in this book has been reached only by means of a series of more or less hard won steps away from the way these concepts are conventionally understood in specialist contexts in hospital medicine – first from fact to value, then from 'disease' to 'illness', and now, in the present section, from 'function' to 'action'. Given the many practical successes of the conventional view, it is right that, although each of these steps was taken for good analytical reasons, each should have been taken cautiously and with care. But it is worth adding in conclusion, that outside the context of hospital medicine, at least the elements of a reverse view would not appear unfamiliar at all. It has already been noted that 'illness' and the evaluative connotations of the medical terms are more prominent in non-specialist than specialist contexts. In chapter 12, similarly, it will be shown that in primary health care – as in general or family practice – a reverse view of the medical concepts is appropriate even in "specialist" contexts. And medical sociologists, indeed, concerned as much with lay as with specialist conceptions of illness and disease, and with what has come to be called "illness behaviour" as much as with illness, have often observed empirically just the same conceptual elements as those identi-

MORAL THEORY AND MEDICAL PRACTICE

fied here analytically. These elements, for example, are explicit in Talcott Parsons' now classical definition of the "sick role" – a role that is, *inter alia*, "undesirable" and one from which one cannot escape by "act of decision or will" (1951). They also emerge clearly, along (as we should expect) with elements of the conventional view, from David Lockyer's detailed inter-view studies (1981, in Ch. 5 for example). Thus the distinctive contribution up to this point of the analysis presented in this book should be understood not so much as demonstrating these elements as ordering and connecting them afresh.

8
Mental illness

We are now ready to pick up the traces of chapter 5. That chapter, it will be recalled, took the form of a progress report on the reverse-view analysis developed in part II. What was found was that although that part had been concerned mainly with 'physical illness', none the less, measured against the two requirements set down at the end of chapter 1, a number of significant steps had already been taken towards a generalization of the analysis from 'physical illness' to 'mental illness'. In this chapter, drawing on the further development of the analysis in chapters 6 and 7 the generalization will be completed.

Requirement 1

The first requirement set down at the end of chapter 1 was that a general concept, 'illness', distinct from the particular, 'physical illness', be demonstrated. The principal contribution of the reverse view developed in part II towards satisfying this requirement was, as it was put in chapter 5, to uncouple the analysis from physical phenomena – 'illness', according to a reverse view, being logically prior to 'disease', rather than vice versa; and illnesses, unlike diseases, being constituted typically, though not exclusively, by feelings and sensations, such as pain, which are (ordinarily thought of as) mental rather than physical phenomena.

This uncoupling process has in effect been taken a step further in this section. For the analysis of 'illness' which has now been developed is in terms, essentially, of 'intention'; and intentions, more securely even than feelings and sensations, are (ordinarily thought of as) mental rather than physical phenomena. But now notice this. The analysis of 'illness' is in terms not just of 'intention' but of ' "intentional" doing' (latent within ' "ordinary" doing'). And the things people do are not limited to the things they do as doing involves their bodies, but include things they do as doing involves their minds. That is to say, people's actions are not limited to things like raising their arms or reaching for books, as in chapter 7, but include things like thinking, calculating and remembering. So that here, in actions being both bodily and mental, is the germ at least, not merely of a generalization of our analysis, but, recalling the caveat noted in chapter 1, of a generalization in the required direction.

But it is really more than just a germ. For all the main ingredients of the analysis of actions like arm raising, in the first third or so of chapter 7, are there also as ingredients of 'mental action'. Thus, (1) mental actions, like bodily actions, as things people do, are distinguished from things that are done or happen to them – compare, for example, 'I thought' and 'I remembered' with 'I was made to think' and 'I was reminded'; and consider the latter not just as everyday responses to encouragement or command but as the results of, say, hypnosis or of propaganda. (2) Mental actions are defined in part by the mental activities performed, but in part also by the purposes for which they are performed – the purpose for which I recall the price of something, for example, is a (logically) necessary part of the specification of that which I am doing in recalling it. (3) Mental action can be (roughly) subdivided into a hierarchy of some more and some less full or complete senses of 'do', according to the extent to which the performer's purpose enters fully into the specification of that which is done – compare here the more or less automatic recall of information involved in starting one's car with the intentional recall of a difficult poem. Yet, (4) mental actions, no less than bodily actions, as everyday things that we ordinarily do, are things that we just get on and do. Hence, it is only when we have cause to reflect on our ordinary mental actions that we find latent within them the components of the full sense(s) of 'do'; such cause being given most commonly and most powerfully, as in the case of our ordinary bodily actions, by difficulties of an external kind, that is to say, by obstruction and/or opposition –

thus, I may have to perform "intentionally" (with my purpose "firmly before my mind") even the most ordinary of mental actions, such as a simple calculation, if I am distracted or disturbed.

There are differences between mental actions and bodily actions, of course. But these are perhaps not so profound as at first sight they appear. This is particularly so in respect of not doing as distinct from doing – the "negative" as distinct from the "positive" case (cf. again chapter 7). It may seem that, compared with not doing most bodily things, there is a difficulty – almost a logical difficulty – in the way of not doing certain mental things. To not-move one's arm one simply keeps it still. But to not-think a particular thought might seem to involve thinking about not thinking it, and hence thinking it after all. Or not remembering something might seem to involve remembering not to remember it, and hence remembering it after all. However, closer inspection shows that mental not-doing and bodily not-doing are really essentially similar. For to not-move one's arm by keeping it still is really to not-do one thing by (in the sense of the word defined here) doing something else. And this "doing something else" is also what is involved in not-thinking and not-remembering things. In order to not-think a particular thought or to not-recall a particular memory, one has to think about or recall something else; or distract oneself in some other way. It is this "doing something else", then, which is implied by such common injunctions as "forget all about it".

'Mental action' and 'bodily action', both negative and positive, are thus closely similar conceptually. And indeed, although they have been spoken of here as though they were quite distinct, in fact, as we saw in chapter 7, most of the things people ordinarily do involve elements of both. For all these reasons, therefore, it seems that 'mental action' and 'bodily action' may well be species of the same general concept of 'action'; the implication being that if 'mental illness' is derived from 'mental action' in the way that 'physical illness' has been found to be derived from 'bodily action', then 'mental illness' and 'physical illness' – or, more appropriately now, '*bodily*' illness – may well be species of the required general concept of 'illness'.

That 'mental illness' *is* so derived has still to be established. But the onus of proof now rests firmly with the sceptics, with those who, in the debate about 'mental illness' outlined in chapter 1, are against the concept rather with those who are for it. All the ingredients being available, the operative question is, not whether mental illness exists, but why it should not exist. Though mark you, even if 'mental illness' is derived from 'mental action', the sceptical position is still just tenable; for this position is not that the concept of 'mental illness' is not employed – of course, it is – but rather that the concept, although employed, is invalid. The sceptic, therefore, while acknowledging the derivation of 'mental illness' from 'mental action', could simply deny the validity of this derivation. He could argue that notwithstanding the similarities between 'mental action' and 'bodily action', it is by some feature(s) peculiar to 'bodily action' that the derivation of 'bodily illness' from it is validated; and further, that if we have been led by the similarities between 'mental action' and 'bodily action' to derive 'mental illness' from 'mental action', then we have been *mis*led.

So there is no short way with scepticism even now. The sceptical position is to be met (or not), as it was in part met in chapter 5, only by explaining, in terms now of our proposed general concept of 'illness', both the similarities and the differences between 'mental illness' and 'bodily illness'. And this leads to the second of the two requirements set out in chapter 1.

Requirement 2

This second requirement, then, was that in proceeding by generalization from 'bodily illness' to 'mental illness', both the similarities and the differences between them should be explained, rather than just ignored or explained away. In chapter 5, however, the contribution of our reverse-view analysis towards satisfying this requirement was made by way of direct comparison rather than by way of generalization. Not, it is true, by way of a tendentious comparison, a comparison of the (misuse of the paradigm argument) kind so commonly adopted in the literature (chapter 1). On the contrary, the comparison developed in chapter 5 was entirely neutral with regard to the question of the validity of the concept of 'mental illness'. But it was a comparison all the same.

Now, though, having taken the argument that much further, the ground has been better prepared for a generalization of the analysis. However, the form of this generalization will have to be somewhat more complicated than anticipated. In chapter 1, the generalization proposed was to be something along the lines of simply measuring various putative examples of mental illness against whatever general concept of 'illness' might eventually be defined. But in chapter 7, in proceeding from 'illness constituted by movement' to 'illness constituted by pain' – itself a mini-generalization – we found that the many similarities between these two kinds of illness could be explained in terms of their common (logical) origins in 'action'. However, even between these two kinds of physical illness there were differences. And these were found to go back to the differences in the ways in which their constituents (movement and pain respectively) were built into the structure of our actions in the first place. In this chapter, then, the form of the larger generalization from 'bodily illness' to 'mental illness' will owe as much to chapter 7 as chapter 1. We will be seeking to explain the similarities between 'mental illness' and 'bodily illness' in terms of their (proposed) common origins in the experience of failure of ' "ordinary" doing', and the differences between them in terms of differences in the ways in which the phenomena by which they are respectively constituted are built into the structure of our actions generally.

Similarities

In chapter 5 the points made on behalf of 'mental illness' were presented under this second requirement somewhat defensively. This was due, no doubt, to the influence of the conventional form of paradigm argument from 'bodily illness'. Thus, echoing Szasz-style scepticism, it was said of the evaluative connotations of 'mental illness', that 'bodily illness', *too*, does have evaluative connotations; and that, if these are less marked on the whole than those of 'mental illness', well, this is at any rate not *prejudicial* to 'mental illness'. Now, however, with a general concept of 'illness' before us, it can be seen, on the contrary, that if a defence is required at all, it is a defence not of 'mental illness' for its more marked evaluative connotations but of 'bodily illness' for its less marked evaluative connotations. For the general concept, 'illness', being derived from 'failure of "ordinary" doing', is itself an evaluative concept. Further, this (conceptually important) point about 'illness' is one which 'mental illness', with its more marked evaluative connotations, reveals, but 'bodily illness', with its less marked evaluative connotations, actually conceals. So that here, following chapter 1, and contrary to the conventional view, it is 'mental illness' rather than 'bodily illness' which is most like 'illness'.

This (as it were) revelatory character of 'mental illness' is the key to this subsection. For what will be found is that 'mental illness' reveals, where 'bodily illness' conceals, not only the evaluative nature of 'illness' but also its (logical) origins in 'action'. Indeed, each of the elements of the analysis of 'bodily illness' which in chapter 7 had to be dragged more or less reluctantly to the surface of that concept, are already there, out in the open as it were, on the surface of 'mental illness'. So in the case of 'mental illness' all that is required for the demonstration of these elements, and hence for the demonstration of a series of at least qualitative similarities between it and 'bodily illness' (over and above their common evaluative natures), is direct inspection of the psychiatric nosology. It is these qualitative similarities that will be explained in this subsection, leaving the corresponding quantitative differences between 'mental illness' and 'body illness' – that is, the greater visibility of each of the elements of our chapter 7 analysis in 'mental illness' than in 'bodily illness' – for the next subsection.

Consider first, then, the first of the two distinctions introduced at the start of chapter 7: namely, that between illness as something wrong with a person and things that are done or happen to that person. This distinction is not too deeply buried even in the case of 'bodily illness'. For although it is only implicit in the ordinary definitions of most bodily illnesses, and although its recognition in the case of 'bodily illness' thus requires a moment's philosophical reflection, none the less it comes out explicitly in the ordinary distinction (noted in chapter 7) between bodily illness and conditions such as bodily injuries or wounds or trauma. In the case of 'mental illness', however, the distinction comes out explicitly in both. As with bodily illness, it comes out in the ordinary distinction between mental illness and mental injuries or wounds or trauma. Thus we speak of being "wounded emotionally", of "psychological trauma" and so on. And though, analogously with their bodily counterparts, there are contingent – and indeed logical – links between mental illness and conditions of this latter kind, they are certainly not logically interchangeable. But the distinction also comes out in the ordinary definitions of (at least certain) mental illnesses. This is clear, for example, in the ICD-9, the World Health Organization's "Ninth Revision of the International Classification of Diseases" (World Health Organization, 1978). There, among "neurotic illnesses" (ICD-9 category 300), 'anxiety state' (300.1) is defined, *inter alia*, as " . . . manifestations of anxiety, not attributable to real danger . . . "; 'phobic state' (300.2) as an " . . . intense dread of certain objects or specific situations which would not normally have that effect . . . "; 'neurotic depression' (300.4) as depression which, though " . . . usually recognisably (ensuing) on a distressing experience (is) disproportionate . . . "; and 'hypochondriasis' (300.7) as " . . . excessive concern with one's health . . . ". Moreover, even among 'psychotic illnesses' (290-9), in some respects closest to physical illness (see chapter 10), the manic type of "manic-depressive psychosis" (296.0) is defined as a state " . . . of elation or excitement out of keeping with the patient's circumstances . . . ". Of course, in calling up observations of ordinary usage in this way, we must remember what can and what cannot be made of them (cf. chapter 1). Taken in isolation, these five fragments of definitions "prove" nothing. For, as they stand, they are susceptible of different interpretations. Indeed, there is evidence to suggest that the authors of ICD-9 themselves might wish to interpret them differently from the way in which they have been interpreted here (see also chapter 9). But taken in context, together with everything that has been and has yet to be said in this book, they are consistent with, and to a small degree they also illumine, the general theory which is now developing. Moreover, as explicit manifestations of the distinction between mental illness and things that are done or happen to people, they represent only the tip of a large if mainly implicit iceberg. As with most bodily illnesses, the distinction is often too self-evident, too taken for granted, for explicit mention. But it is there, nevertheless. The patient with a hysterical (that is, psychogenic) paraplegia (ICD-9 300.5), for example, no more than his organically paralysed counterpart, is not prevented from moving his legs by some external obstruction and/or opposition. Likewise, the obsessive-compulsive patient (300.3), perhaps interminably washing his hands, is not compelled (by anyone else, *vide infra*) to do so. The alcoholic and the drug addict (304) are not force-fed their alcohol or their drugs. The anorexic (307.1) is not denied food. And the dement (290) is not prevented from remembering things, or from knowing what time it is or where he or she is, by external distraction or obstruction.

Interestingly, however, in cases of the latter kind, if the first of the two initial chapter 7 distinctions is left mainly implicit, the second – that between illness as something wrong with someone and things that the person does – is often made explicit. We will come to the reasons for this, and indeed for the converse often being true of conditions (like anxiety states) of the kind noted in the paragraph before last, in the next subsection. But for now, notice, at least, just how explicit the second distinction can be. In ICD-9 again, it comes out clearly in the distinction between the (presumed) disease alcoholism or dipsomania (two ICD-9 synonyms for its category 303, the "alcohol-dependence syndrome") and mere drunkenness (an ICD-9 synonym for 305.0, "non-dependent abuse of alcohol"). According to ICD-9 the alcoholic experiences "a compulsion to take alcohol", whereas the drunk takes it on his "own initiative", the implication being that the alcoholic's drinking, being something he is compelled to do, is not (like the drunk's) something that he (in the full sense of the word) does. ICD-9 employs the notion of 'compulsion' in a similar manner in its definitions of drug addiction (304) and obsessive-compulsive neurosis (300.3). Furthermore, although it describes hysterical neuroses (300.1) as "produced by" motives, it says that these are "motives of which the patient is unaware". So the hysteric, too, is not (in the full sense of the word) doing something.

'Mental illness', therefore, according to the evidence of ordinary usage, is like 'bodily illness' to the extent that it is subject to the same two initial distinctions: like 'bodily illness', it is distinguished both from things that are done or happen to people and from things that they do. Again, though, it is important not to make too much of this. Our objective, here, is simply to mark the qualitative similarities between 'mental illness' and 'bodily illness'. There is no question, on the strength of these similarities alone, of attempting to prove that 'mental illness' is derived from 'mental action', let alone of proving that it is derived from it in the way that (as was suggested in chapter 7) 'bodily illness' is derived from 'bodily action'. However, it is of course true that support for the belief that 'mental illness' is so derived is provided by these similarities. For in chapter 7 it was the fact that 'bodily illness' is subject to these two distinctions that led to an examination of the sense of 'do' in which people ordinarily do things, and thus to the derivation of 'bodily illness' from the experience of failure of ' "ordinary" doing' in the absence of obstruction and/or opposition. And here, now, is 'mental illness', subject, apparently, to the same two distinctions. And not only that. For the sense of 'do' in which the mentally ill patient – the hysteric, the obsessive-compulsive neurotic, the alcoholic – is *not* doing something, turns out to be in all relevant respects closely similar to the sense of 'do' from which our chapter 7 analysis of 'bodily illness' was derived.

Thus, in the first place, and significantly, the things that the mentally ill patient is not doing are, as they were for the bodily ill patient, "everyday things that people ordinarily just get on and do" (cf. chapter 7); moving their arms and legs, remembering (common or garden) things, finding their way about (familiar) places and so on. Indeed, 'mental illness' brings out rather well the fact, noted under Requirement 1 in this chapter, that ordinary mental doing is like ordinary bodily doing in covering both the negative and the positive case. In chapter 7, this property of ' "ordinary" doing' allowed the constraint introduced at the start of that chapter to be satisfied: namely, that whatever analysis of 'illness' is proposed, it must cover, as ' "ordinary" doing' covers, the negative as well as the positive case – the paralytic who is unable to move as well as the choreic and the athetotic who cannot *not* move. And so it is here, and more strikingly, for mental illness. The dement, analogously with the paralytic, cannot recall things. Neither can the hysteric – though, as we saw in the paragraph before last, there is an important sense in which the hysteric is actually refusing to recall, rather than simply being unable to do so. But the obsessional neurotic, on the other hand, plagued with obsessional images, say, is more like the choreic or the athetotic. He cannot *not* recall things. It is no good telling him, as (under Requirement 1 above) we were ready to tell anyone else, to forget all about it. This is just what he, the obsessional neurotic, cannot do. His obsessions, resist them as he may, come back relentlessly into his mind. Indeed, Wing and his colleagues, in the glossary to their carefully standardized diagnostic interview, the "Present State Examination" (or PSE, see Wing *et al.*, 1974), make this ineffective resistance the central feature of that whole range of both obsessive (= mental) and compulsive (= bodily) doings by which the obsessive-compulsive neurotic may be beset. As it is put in the PSE (symptoms 44, 45 and 46, p. 157), the obsessional neurotic patient recognizes that his constant recalling of certain images – or his thinking of certain thoughts or his repeating of certain sequences of letters or numbers or his endless checking or his arranging and rearranging objects in set patterns or his perpetual washing or whatever – is all quite "senseless and (he) tries to resist it but cannot". So an obsessional symptom is like a very bad case of getting a tune "stuck in one's head".

In the first place, then, the sense of 'do' in which the mentally ill patient is not doing something is the same as that in which the bodily ill patient is not doing something; it is that of

' "ordinary" doing', and "ordinary" doing as covering both the negative and the positive case. But in the second place, and more important still, the components of these two kinds of "ordinary" doing – "ordinary" mental doing and "ordinary" bodily doing – are the same. They are indeed just those noted as components of "mental action" under Requirement 1 in this chapter. And in this subsection, under Requirement 2, it has been the absence of one or more of these components which has made it possible to say that the mentally ill patient is not doing something in the full sense of that word. Thus, the ICD-9 alcoholic, to the extent that he is "compelled" to drink, is not serving his *own purposes* (as it was put in chapter 7). Whereas the ICD-9 drunk, acting on his "own initiative", is. Similarly, the ICD-9 hysteric, although acting from his own "motives" is not acting *intentionally* because he is not "aware" of these motives. This is brought out further in the American Psychiatric Association's "Diagnostic and Statistical Manual of Mental Disorders" (or DSM-III, American Psychiatric Association, 1980), a classification intended (DSM-III, p. 2) as a further development of ICD-9. For in DSM-III, hysterical symptoms (300.11) are allowed to serve what are described as "conscious" as well as "unconscious needs" – so-called secondary and primary gain respectively (DSM-III, p. 244). But in both cases, such symptoms are said, none the less, not to be "under *voluntary control*". Furthermore, it is on just this point that in DSM-III the symptoms of a hysterical neurosis proper are distinguished from those of simulated illness, DSM-III's "factitious disorder", disorder which is "not real, genuine or natural" (DSM-III, p. 285). For in DSM-III, the symptoms of a factitious disorder, which may be bodily or mental, are described as being unlike those of a hysterical disorder, precisely in being "under voluntary control" (DSM-III, p. 285). However, even factitious disorder does not amount to true "malingering" as a condition "not attributable to a mental disorder" at all (DSM-III, p. 331). For the "acts" by which the symptoms of a factitious disorder are produced, although variously described as being "purposeful", "intentional" and "voluntary", are still said to have a "compulsive quality" (DSM-III, p. 285). So that, according to DSM-III, the patient with a factitious disorder, unlike the true malingerer, is "unable to refrain" from simulating illness; which is to say, again in the terminology of chapter 7, that the patient with a factitious disorder lacks that important additional component of the full sense of 'do', "*self control*".

'Mental illness' and 'bodily illness' are thus similar in a number of conceptually significant respects. Both are subject to the same two initial distinctions, from things that are done or happen to people and from things that they do. And the sense of 'do' implied in the second of these distinctions is ' "ordinary" doing', ' "ordinary" doing' as covering the negative as well as the positive case, and made up of the same basic components. As has several times been said, the mere demonstration of these similarities does not in itself amount to proof that 'mental illness' is derived from 'mental action' as 'bodily illness' is derived from 'bodily action'. But these similarities are at least fully consistent with this being so. Indeed, they are explained by it being so. And extensive as they are, it is not easy to see how else they could be explained.

Differences

As the revelatory character of 'mental illness' was the key to the last subsection – 'mental illness' revealing, where 'bodily illness' conceals, the origins of 'illness' in 'action' – so the *reason* for its revelatory character is the key to this subsection.

In chapter 5 the differences between 'mental illness' and 'bodily illness' (and between 'mental disease' and 'bodily disease') were interpreted in terms of differences in the properties, both empirical and evaluative, of their respective illness constituents. In particular, the more overtly evaluative connotations of 'mental illness' compared with 'bodily illness' were shown to be due to the criteria by which mental-illness constituents (like anxiety) are evaluated being on the whole more variable than the criteria by which bodily-illness constituents (like pain) are evaluated. In the terms of the present chapter, therefore, it can now be said that the reason why the evaluative nature of 'illness' is revealed more by 'mental illness' than by 'bodily illness', is that the value judgement expressed by 'illness' is on the whole more problematic – and hence more eye-catching – when it is used of mental-illness constituents than when it is used of bodily-illness constituents. And much the same will be found in this subsection to be true for the origins of 'illness' in 'action'. For what will be found is that the reason why the origins of 'illness' in 'action' are revealed more by 'mental illness' than by 'bodily illness', is that these origins are on the whole more problematic (and hence more eye-catching) in respect of mental-illness constituents than they are in respect of bodily-illness constituents. As in chapter 5, therefore, so also in this chapter, the differences between 'mental illness' and 'bodily illness' will be found to be (or to be derived from) differences in the properties of the phenomena by which they are respectively constituted. And 'mental illness' will thus turn out not to be prejudiced but rather to be endorsed by the differences between it and 'bodily illness'.

In this chapter, however, with regard to the origins of 'illness' in 'action', matters are bound to be more complicated than they were in chapter 5. In chapter 5, in respect of the evaluative nature of 'illness', only one underlying property of the constituents of illness had to be considered – namely, the wider variation in the criteria by which mental- as opposed to bodily-illness constituents are evaluated. But here the underlying properties that must be considered are various. For different illness constituents – bodily and mental – are incorporated differently into the structure of our actions: movement, as we saw in chapter 7, differently from pain; thought and memory, as in this chapter, similarly to movement; and anxiety, perhaps, similarly to pain; but thought and memory, in turn, differently from hunger; and so on. Hence, for each of these different ways in which different illness constituents may be incorporated into the structure of our actions, different problems can arise at different stages and for different reasons.

A complete explanation of the tendency of 'mental illness' to reveal the origins of 'illness' in 'action', by an argument parallel to the explanation in chapter 5 of its tendency to reveal the evaluative nature of 'illness', would thus amount to a large undertaking. It would be a large philosophical undertaking because it would involve exploring separately for each illness constituent the way(s) in which it may be incorporated into the structure of our actions, the problems which can arise, and the reflections of these problems in the failures of ' "ordinary" doing' by which (if the analysis presented here is right) the illnesses constituted by it are defined. It would also be a large clinical undertaking, because the data upon which the philosophical explorations would rely would have to be drawn from detailed studies of ordinary usage, going well beyond the mainly literary sources utilized in this chapter, into actual clinical practice.

In this subsection, therefore, rather than tilting at completeness, we will examine in more detail just one of the conditions mentioned in the last subsection – namely, alcoholism. Even so, the objective will not be a complete or final account of the definition of 'alcoholism'. All that will be attempted will be to explain the observations made in the last subsection: why it should be that the "illness-versus-done-by" distinction appears explicitly in clinical definitions of 'alcoholism', the condition being defined in both ICD-9 and DSM-III in terms of 'compulsion'; and why it is that alcoholism is in this respect similar to some mental illnesses (such as drug addiction, hysteria and obsessive-compulsive neurosis), yet different from others (such as anxiety and depressive neuroses, in the clinical definitions of which it is the "illness-versus-done-or-happens-to" distinction which is made explicit). These issues will be approached indirectly, by looking first at the features of alcoholism which are conceptually problematic in clinical practice, then at the failure of both conventional and the limited part II reverse-view analyses of 'illness' to explain them, and finally at the explanations which flow from the extended reverse view developed in the present section.

Alcoholism, notoriously perhaps, has not always been thought of as a disease (see, for example, Jellinek, 1960). Nor, even now, is it universally accepted that the alcoholic is ill. Alcoholism is included, as in ICD-9 and DSM-III, in most modern disease classifications. Yet its status as a disease continues to be debated. Furthermore, unlike that of most other mental illnesses, it continues to be debated as much among doctors as among others, and indeed as much among those who otherwise are *for* the concept of 'mental illness' as among those who are *against* it. Thus, Kendell (1979), whose pro-'mental illness' views were considered in chapter 1, has argued against the disease concept of alcoholism in terms strongly reminiscent of the anti-'mental illness' arguments of his opponent, Szasz. He describes the concept as being the result of a "campaign" with a definite historical origin (with Thomas Trotter in 1804), and he says that it has now become "official dogma", which, though it has had some humanitarian consequences, tends to be used as a "convenient excuse" by industry and by politicians, even by patients themselves, in order to avoid tackling the "problem" effectively.

A first conceptually problematic feature of alcoholism in clinical practice is thus the uncertainty – as much among doctors as among others – regarding its disease status. To a first level of approximation, however, there is no mystery about this. Alcoholism is associated clinically with a wide variety of all those non-empirical problems which were found in chapter 1 to be the mainspring of the debate about 'mental illness' generally. Indeed, it is primarily with problems of this kind, with the ethical, medico-legal and especially the political problems associated with alcoholism that Kendell is concerned in his 1979 paper. Furthermore, among specifically conceptual difficulties, the "illness-diagnostic" difficulty introduced right at the start of chapter 1, and in terms of which the uncertain disease status of mental illness generally was explained in chapter 4, is raised by alcoholism in a particularly acute way. The alcoholic, according to the clinical definitions noted in the last subsection, is distinguished diagnostically from the drunk in being under a compulsion to drink. But this distinction, easy as it is to state, is peculiarly difficult to draw. And the difficulty here is not, or not solely or primarily, empirical but conceptual. The difficulty will be examined in more detail in a moment. But it amounts to this: that however well established the facts of a given case are (as to quantity, type, frequency and effects of alcohol consumption and so on), there seems always to be some residual scope for the case to be construed either way, either as a case of being unable to resist the urge to drink (= compulsion = alcoholism) or as a case of simply not resisting it (= no compulsion = drunken-ness).

Moreover, what is at stake here is not just whether the patient is ill or well, but also whether he is (as an alcoholic) ill or (as a drunk) at fault morally. This distinction, between illness and moral fault, is one which is of course implicit in the concept of 'illness' generally (chapter 5). But it is especially close to the surface in the diagnosis of alcoholism − witness in ICD-9 the explicit mention of drunkenness in its differential diagnosis. And this feature of alcoholism, therefore, in addition to bringing an extra edge to the diagnostic difficulties with which it is associated, thus also stands in its own right as a further problematic feature to be explained − and explained consistently with the fact that alcoholism, although similar in this respect to some mental illnesses, is different not only from most bodily illnesses but also from certain other mental illnesses as well. The distinction, for example, between bulimia (illness) and gluttony (moral fault), although always there in principle, is not in practice one which is normally at issue diagnostically. The illness versus moral fault distinction is not clinically problematic here. But contrast this with certain of the so-called disorders of sexual object choice: with fetishism, for example, or homosexuality. The status of these conditions, consistently with the diagnostic problems with which they are associated, has undergone even sharper fluctuations in recent years than has that of alcoholism, not only as between illness and moral fault but also as between both these and normality.

At the heart of the uncertain disease status of alcoholism, therefore, is, as we should expect from our findings in chapters 4 and 5, the "illness-diagnostic" difficulty. And the particular acuteness of this difficulty in this case explains (to the extent that it is consistent with) the disease status of alcoholism being so uncertain. In the terminology of chapter 4, alcoholism is a condition on the edge of the subcategory Id. Yet this being so, conventional medical models of the kind discussed in chapters 2 and 3 provide no insight at all into just why it should be so. Indeed, such models are flatly contradicted by the fact that it is so. For according to such models, alcoholism, far from being only uncertainly a disease, should be paradigmatically so. It is true that there is room for a degree of uncertainty in some of the more naïve medical models – as in the fact, for example, recalling statistical models of 'disease', that the alcoholic, though often drinking more alcohol than others, may, according to Williams and Strauss (1950), actually drink less. But then it is clear already, from what was said in chapter 2, that naïve models of this kind are logically flawed in a number of obvious ways. Nor is there more room for uncertainty in more sophisticated 'dysfunction'-based medical models. For here if anywhere, surely, in the alcoholic's compulsion to drink, there would seem to be a disturbance of function – of the "appetitive" system or the "pleasure–pain"/"reward–punishment" mechanisms underlying learned behaviour and so on – exactly as is required by such models. Moreover, here surely, if anywhere, again as required by such models, there would seem to be a good descriptivist case to be made for the alcoholic's particular compulsion being marked out as a *disturbance* of function (as distinct from the compulsion to drink water when thirsty, say) by reference to essentially factual/scientific criteria; indeed, by reference to just those factual/scientific criteria invoked by Kendell among others in defining the notion of 'mental illness'– namely, reduced life and/or reproductive expectations (c.f. chapter 3).

With alcoholism, however, the limited reverse view developed in part II fares little better than the conventional view. It provides a better general working framework, perhaps. In recognizing the logical priority of 'illness' over 'disease', for example, it clarifies the distinction (which has not always been well maintained in the literature) between alcohol consumption as an illness constituent – as in 'alcoholism' proper – and alcohol consumption as an HDf2-style aetiological differentium of other diseases – as in 'alcoholic cirrhosis', 'alcoholic psychosis' and so on. Then again, in making central, rather than excluding, the evaluative element in the meanings of 'illness' and 'disease', it at least falls into the right conceptual area for an examination of the distinction between alcohol consumption as an illness constituent – as in 'alcoholism' proper – and alcohol consumption as morally delinquent behaviour – as in 'drunkenness'. But despite this better general working framework, the limited reverse view of part II fails in respect of 'alcoholism' when it comes to the particular. The explanation given in chapter 5 for the uncertain disease status of many mental illnesses rested (like that for their more overtly evaluative connotations) on the (psychological) variability of the criteria by which their constituent phenomena are evaluated. This explanation worked well enough for illness constituents such as anxiety and pain; the criteria by which anxiety (a typical mental-illness constituent) is evaluated being more variable than the criteria by which pain (a typical bodily-illness constituent) is evaluated. But, logical considerations notwithstanding, there is not the same psychological scope for variation in the criteria by which alcohol consumption is evaluated. There is some scope, certainly, and more than for pain. But on these grounds the disease status of an illness constituted by alcohol consumption (that is, alcoholism), although less certain than that of an illness constituted by pain (that is, a typical bodily illness), should in turn be *more* certain than that of an illness constituted by anxiety. Yet it is not.

What account of 'alcoholism', then, and of the problems raised by it, is given by the 'action failure'-based analysis of 'illness', the extended reverse view developed in the present section? To see this, it is necessary first to consider more carefully the notion of 'alcoholism', the actual clinical syndrome of "compulsive alcohol consumption". What is involved here? As we have seen, it is not that the alcoholic is compelled by anyone else to drink. The compulsion, such as it is, is from within. But there are different kinds of compulsion even from within. The alcoholic differs, for example, from the epileptic (who in the course of an epileptic fugue may drink large quantities of alcohol) in being compelled by a conscious urge to drink. Then again, the alcoholic differs from the obsessive-compulsive neurotic, in that the urge to drink by which he is compelled is an appetitive urge – that is to say, it is an urge which is experienced not merely as an impulse to drink alcohol, as an obsessional urge would be, but as a desire or craving for it. And this desire or craving in the alcoholic differs from an ordinary desire for a drink in that even if the alcoholic intends to resist it, he is unable to. This is the failure of "ordinary" doing by which, according to the analysis of chapter 7, alcoholism is linked conceptually with other species of illness. The phenomenon by which alcoholism is constituted is thus better thought of not as alcohol consumption as such – as it was described a moment ago – but rather as a desire for alcohol.

Now consider what is involved in making a diagnosis of alcoholism, so defined. What is likely to be problematic about this diagnosis? Well, first off there is the attribution of intentions. In this, of course, as far as it goes, and tricky as it may be, the diagnosis of alcoholism is in principle no different from that of any other illness. ' "Ordinary" doing', as defined in chapter 7, is made up in part of intentions, the attribution of which is therefore necessary to the attribution of *failure* of ' "ordinary" doing'. But in the case of alcoholism, as defined clinically, the particular intention which is attributed, being an intention to resist the desire for alcohol, is an intention in respect of a desire. And with intentions of *this* kind, there is special scope for difficulty. For desires are closer to intentions conceptually than are many of the other illness constituents so far considered. In particular, both are species of "wants": to desire something is to want it (though one may want other things more); to intend to do something is to want to do it (if not for its own sake, at least for the sake of something else). So here, at the very least, is an opportunity for confusion, between the wanting of desiring and the wanting of intending, which is simply not there in respect of illness constituents such as movement, pain, anxiety, sadness, remembering and thinking.

This is not to say that the two kinds of wanting are indistinguishable. It is to say only that there is a potential difficulty in distinguishing them. And if we now consider the way in which intentions are attributed, we will see how this potential is in fact realized in the diagnosis of alcoholism, and thus how the difficulties to which the diagnosis is subject are generated.

In attributing intentions, information of at least two kinds is usually available: information about the person to whom the intention in question is to be attributed and information about people's intentions generally. Both sorts of information are derived in part from what people say, in part from what they do, on the given occasion and also in general. These different sources of information carry different weights: on the whole what people do carries more weight than what they say; and what the person in question does carries more weight than what people in general do in similar circumstances. This is so because people normally do things intentionally, intention being latent in ' "ordinary" doing'. Indeed, for something which someone does to be taken to be done *other* than intentionally, special circumstances have to be invoked – accident, impediment, incapacity, inattention, compulsion and so on. People, that is to say, are taken to do things intentionally unless proved otherwise.

However, the things people do are a mark, generally, of what they want. So the things people do can be a mark as much of what they "want = desire" as of what they "want = intend". Thus, although the attribution of any intention whatsoever may be subject to difficulty (the information which is available being insufficient, say, or contradictory), the attribution of intentions in respect of desires is subject to the further difficulty that at least half the information which is available (that which relates to what people do) is necessarily ambiguous.

Now this difficulty, though unavoidable in principle, can in practice usually be ignored. For usually the information which is available in attributing intentions in respect of desires, all points the same way. When this is so, and when there are no special circumstances, it will be assumed that what is done is done, as anything else is ordinarily done, intentionally. In respect of a desire for a drink, for example, if I *say* that I would like (that is want = desire) a drink and *have* one, then, it being assumed that what I do (have a drink) I do intentionally, the intention which is attributed to me will be to satisfy my desire for a drink. This is the simplest case. Another more complicated case would be if I say that I would like a drink and then do not have one. But even in this case, there is usually additional information available, which, together with the assumption that what I do I do intentionally, will point to my intention being *not* to satisfy my desire for a drink for the sake of some further thing that I want more – for example, to avoid a breathalyser test or a hangover, or to keep a clear head. I may actually evince these further intentions, which would be one piece of additional information. Or more information may be provided by the situation as a whole. In particular, it may be that the consequences of my not having a drink in the situation in question are consequences that *people generally* would intentionally entertain.

But in the case of alcoholism, all this breaks down because the information which is available points different ways. On the one hand, what the alcoholic *says* is that although he very much wants (= desires) alcohol, so much so that he is "compelled" to drink (cf. ICD-9), none the less what he wants (= intends) is not to drink. His intentions, even as expressed, may be mixed, of course, and often are. But that his intention is indeed not to drink is borne out to some extent by the consequences of his drinking – namely, adverse psychological, social, medical and financial consequences. These are consequences that people generally would not intentionally entertain. Indeed, Keller (1960) draws implicitly on just this point in making his key criterion of the relevance of an "ill effect" to the diagnosis of alcoholism whether the individual would be "expected to reduce his drinking (or give it up) in order to avoid it". On the other hand, however, what the alcoholic actually *does*, is to go on drinking. As we have seen, this could, and in the absence of special circumstances normally would, be taken to point to it being his intention to do so. The special circumstance which is claimed by the alcoholic is compulsion, of course. But this being an internal, desire-driven compulsion, the only external evidence for it is his continued drinking. This *could* be taken to point to his want (= desire) for alcohol being so strong that his wanting (= intending) not to drink in order to avoid the consequences is overwhelmed by it. But equally it could, and normally would, be taken to point to his want (= desire) for alcohol being so strong that he wants (= intends) to go on drinking *despite* the consequences. And on this ambiguity of interpretation the matter has to rest. Either the alcoholic's desire is irresistible, or it is not resisted. If it is irresistible, he is ill; if not, he is a drunk. There is no way to decide finally between these alternatives on the information which is available. Hence there is always room for the diagnosis to be construed either way; hence the particular acuteness of the conceptual difficulty to which this diagnosis is subject in practice.

This difficulty, as one clinically problematic feature of alcoholism, can thus be derived from an underlying difficulty of a general kind in the attribution of intentions in respect of desires. Explanations for the other clinically problematic features of alcoholism now follow readily.

First, there is the particular prominence in respect of alcoholism of the illness versus moral-fault distinction, described earlier as an extra edge to the diagnostic difficulty in this case. This distinction hinges, as noted in chapter 7, on the attribution of intentions. Among things people do, it is in general only those that they do intentionally which are held morally praiseworthy or blameworthy. But 'illness', according to the argument of chapter 7, is derived from *failure* of ' "ordinary" (and hence intentional) doing'. In the case of alcoholism, therefore, the illness versus moral-fault distinction will be difficult to make for the same reason that the diagnosis is difficult generally – that is because of the underlying difficulty in attributing intentions in respect of desires. But the distinction is important, and therefore prominent clinically, only to the extent that the particular desire by which alcoholism is constituted is itself important, and hence prominent, in morality. It is the "lusts of the flesh", as it were, which are showing through here. So, it is because the distinction between illness and moral fault is difficult to draw here, that alcoholism is put at issue diagnostically in respect of this distinction; and it is because the distinction is morally important that the diagnostic issue is clinically prominent.

Second, and tied in with this, is the fact that alcoholism is in this respect similar to some mental illness (disorders of sexual object choice) but different from others (bulimia). If it is the "lusts of the flesh" which are showing through in the case of alcoholism, it is similar lusts which are showing through in the prominence of the illness versus moral-fault distinction in the case of disorders of sexual object choice (such as fetishism). Correspondingly, to the extent that the distinction between bulimia and gluttony is not clinically prominent, this is because, although the difficulty of attributing intentions in respect of desires is present in principle, gluttony is not taken to be a very serious vice currently; though, interestingly, bulimics themselves usually feel guilty about their bingeing. (Of course, the *disease* bulimia, as distinct from the symptom, is defined in part by pathological eating behaviour, in part by associated signs and symptoms. It is the definition of the symptom – eating behaviour as a constituent of illness – that we are considering here.)

A third clinically problematic feature is the uncertain disease status of alcoholism. As noted earlier this follows straightforwardly from the illness-diagnostic difficulties to which alcoholism is subject. Because of these difficulties, alcoholism, while falling into the chapter 4 category 'I', is only on the edge of the sub-category 'Id'. And the particular acuteness of the illness-diagnostic difficulty in the case of alcoholism correlates with the particular uncertainty of its disease status. A hangover, by the way, one of the examples of "illness-not-disease" noted in chapter 2, is even further from Id, being a consequence of alcohol excess of *any* kind (non-compulsive as well as compulsive), and hence more so than alcoholism something one *does* (to oneself).

In sum, then, each of the clinically problematic features of the concept of 'alcoholism' can be derived from an underlying difficulty in the attribution of intentions in respect of desires. It is this underlying difficulty which is at the root of the diagnostic difficulty with which alcoholism is associated. This diagnostic difficulty, in turn, combined with the moral significance attached to drunkenness, explains the prominence of the illness versus moral-fault distinction in respect of alcoholism. And these two features together, both being illness-diagnostic difficulties, explain the uncertain status of alcoholism as a disease.

The argument of this subsection, therefore, has run as anticipated, parallel with that of the corresponding subsection of chapter 5. Alcoholism has been shown to reveal the origins of 'illness' in 'action' essentially because these origins are, in the case of alcoholism, problematic. There is clearly much more to be said in respect of alcoholism, both clinically and philosophically; and alcoholism has been considered here only by way of illustration. But it can be seen by analogy that it should be possible to develop similar arguments for other mental illnesses. The underlying problems will differ, and, corresponding with differences in their clinical definitions, it is to be expected that some of these problems will be (as with alcoholism) in the "illness versus done by" distinction by which 'illness' is defined, whereas others will be in the "illness versus done or happens to" distinction. And to the extent that this turns out to be so, the differences in this respect between 'mental illness' generally and 'bodily illness' will have been explained, as the similarities between them were explained in the last subsection, in terms of the general concept of 'illness' derived in chapter 7.

PRACTICAL APPLICATIONS

Part IV

9
Diagnosis

Up to now our reverse-view analysis has been developed mainly under the first outcome criterion adopted in chapter 1, namely, its ability to explain and clarify ordinary usage. In this part, under the second outcome criterion, some of its practical applications will be examined. As we will see, the two main areas of clinical activity, diagnosis and treatment, are closely related conceptually. For convenience, however, they will be considered separately; diagnosis in this chapter, treatment in the next. In both chapters it will be mainly psychological medicine that we will have in mind, since it is here, rather than in physical medicine, that the non-empirical clinical problems towards which philosophical analysis is principally directed are most evident. The implications of the analysis for medicine generally will be outlined in chapter 12.

Diagnosis, as touched on in chapter 4, can be thought of essentially as deciding what is wrong with someone. In most branches of physical medicine, whatever practical difficulties are presented by an individual case, a decision about what is wrong can be made within a classification of things wrong which is very largely settled both among different health care professionals (doctors, nurses, social workers, administrators) and internationally. In psychological medicine, however, despite much progress in recent years, diagnosis remains hampered by the lack of a satisfactory and generally accepted classification. It is here that a reverse-view analysis of the medical concepts could prove helpful.

The potential contribution of a reverse-view analysis in this respect is best seen in its historical context. Modern classifications of mental disorders, such as the ICD-9 and DSM-III, have their origins in the mid-nineteenth century. Until then, although (over some 3000 years) classifications of mental disorders had been plentiful enough (Menninger, 1963), they had been developed mainly by philosophers (including Plato and Kant) or by physicians (such as Thomas Willis) as part of the development of general classifications of disease. But now, with the growth in importance of lunatic asylums in the rapidly expanding European and American cities of the industrial revolution, there appeared for the first time a generation of doctors, men in the tradition of Pinel and Esquirol, who specialized in and had detailed clinical experience of mental disorders. From the first, though, the difficulties inherent in the classification of these disorders were apparent. Far from a consensus emerging from this new breed of experts, it seemed that as Kendell put it (1975b, p. 87), "every self-respecting alienist, and certainly every professor, had his own classification". It is true that the main outlines of our modern classifications were present from an early stage. They had indeed stabilized essentially in their current form by 1899, with the publication of the sixth edition of Emil Kraepelin's *Lehrbuch*. Even so, and despite the efforts of a number of international committees, progress towards agreement on the particular disease categories which should be recognized within these outlines had to wait for the formation of the World Health Organization in 1948. In fact, one of the very first acts of WHO was to publish an international classification of diseases, the ICD-6 (WHO, 1948), based on the fifth edition of the then well-established International List of Causes of Death. Though the main effect of ICD-6, from the point of view of psychological medicine, was to bring out the extent of the differences and disagreements which remained, since, although it gained wide acceptance generally, its psychiatric section (chapter v) was adopted by only five member states. It was only with ICD-8 (WHO, 1967), a classification based on new principles laid down in a report commissioned by WHO from the English psychiatrist Erwin Stengel (1959), that broad international agreement in this area was finally achieved. The current ICD-9, published in 1978, and, in turn, the DSM-III (1980), are both derived from ICD-8.

This historical progress, although prompted by social changes, has been moulded throughout largely by the conventional view. Thus, psychological medicine, driven mainly by empirical clinical needs, has followed physical medicine in developing its classifications of "things wrong" on the model of physical-disease categories; categories defined factually to the exclusion of value, and in terms of 'dysfunction' to the exclusion of 'illness'. There have been good reasons for this. The original urge to classify, after all, in the nineteenth century, was prompted by the dramatic advances during that period in the classification of physical diseases made possible by the appearance of the "germ theory" and other medical scientific successes. And many of the classifications of mental disorders produced in both the nineteenth and the first half of the twentieth centuries attempted to follow physical-disease classifications in being aetiologically based. These attempts, as Stengel emphasized in his report, turned out to be premature, a great many of the differences between the rival classifications of the period reflecting (still unresolved) differences of aetiological opinion. Kraepelin's classification, on the other hand, being based on the symptoms and course of mental disorders rather than on theories of their aetiology, was more successful in part because it returned to an earlier stage in the development of physical-disease theory – namely, to the symptomatic, pre-aetiological stage of Sydenham and others in the seventeenth and early eighteenth centuries. And Stengel's main recommendation to the WHO, the one which led to the success of ICD-8, was, in effect, that in the development of the International Classification, Kraepelin's lead should be followed. As a result, the disease categories adopted in ICD-8, unlike those in previous international classifications, were defined largely in terms of symptoms. And this has left psychiatrists free to exploit more fully the empirical methods of scientific psychology in trying to establish a firm descriptive basis for their classifications – on symptoms which are reliably identifiable and on syndromes which are operationally defined (Hempel, 1961) – with consequent improvements which, indeed, are now reflected in ICD-9 and in DSM-III.

The operation of the conventional view in relation to the classification of mental disorders has thus been to excellent effect, especially in recent years. Yet deep difficulties remain.

The ICD, and in the United States the DSM, may have been adopted officially, but their actual use, as classifications within which clinical diagnoses are actually made, has been disappointingly limited. Both classifications have found some application in research: the ICD, with its broadly drawn and internationally acceptable definitions, mainly in large-scale epidemiological surveys, of schizophrenia for example, (Cooper *et al.*, 1972); and the DSM, with its more detailed inclusion and exclusion criteria for individual diseases, in a wide variety of research situations. But even in research there has been a tendency for individual workers to adapt the official classifications to their particular needs, rather than to adopt them as they stand. And in everyday clinical work the impact, especially of the ICD, has been minimal. Kendell (1975b) demonstrated this clearly for ICD-8; two years before its introduction he found that 25 per cent of hospital diagnoses were in ICD terms, two years after its introduction the number had risen only to 27 per cent. Similarly, a glance at any set of ordinary clinical notes will show that the present situation, despite further improvements in ICD-9 and DSM-III, is little better. The broad categories of disorder are there, as they have been almost from the start. But as to individual diseases, the diagnoses that are made remain markedly idiosyncratic. And even in clinical textbooks the official classifications are not often adopted unchanged.

At least in clinical work, therefore, psychological medicine seems not to have moved very far from its original nineteenth-century state of clinical diagnostic individualism. There has been no recent investigation of any comprehensive kind into why this should be so. But given the pragmatic nature of medicine, if the official classifications are not used, this is probably because, despite recent improvements, they are still not particularly useful from a clinical point of view. Clinicians, after all, as Wulff (1976) has emphasized, are concerned with classifications of disease only to the extent that such classifications are indeed useful clinically. And certainly, if one tries to use the current classifications clinically, in making diagnoses, one finds them unduly procrustean in perhaps a majority of cases. That is to say, the clinical facts often have to be pushed or pulled, stretched or squeezed, before "what is wrong" can be accommodated to the categories in the official classifications. According to the conventional view, this is because the scientific foundations of these classifications remain insecure. Thus Kendell (1975b) notes recently renewed pressure for aetiologically based classifications. He argues that this is premature, in the present state of the development of scientific psychiatry, and he says that we should look rather to improved descriptive criteria as the basis of further refinements to our present classifications.

But according to a reverse view of the logical structure of medicine, there is likely to be a good deal more to it than just this. A reverse view of course acknowledges the need for scientific advances of the kind envisaged under the conventional view. Indeed, as we will see in a moment, it actually promotes such advances. But in addition, it suggests, first, that advances of this kind can lead to improvements only in the (important) empirical elements in our classifications; second, that in these classifications there are likely to be, besides these empirical elements, largely unrecognized (though equally important) non-empirical elements; and third, that improvements with regard to such non-empirical elements could well make as decisive a contribution to the clinical usefulness of our classifications as improvements in their empirical elements. The reverse view developed here, after all, has come out of an analysis of the conceptual structure of medicine made necessary by the growing importance in recent years of *non*-empirical clinical problems (cf. chapter 1). And right at the very start of this analysis it was noted that not all diagnostic problems, at least in psychological medicine, are of a conventional empirical kind. Hence there is a good *prima-facie* case for supposing that a reverse-view classification of mental disorders, in which the non-empirical elements are developed equally alongside the empirical – evaluation alongside description, 'illness' alongside 'disease', and the analysis of 'illness' in terms of 'action failure' alongside the analysis of 'disease' in terms of 'dysfunction' – there is a good *prima-facie* case for supposing that such a classification would go further than the present conventional-view classifications towards satisfying clinical diagnostic needs.

The full development of a reverse-view classification, set out in detail, would require a considerable ongoing research effort, both clinical and philosophical, an effort no less than that which has gone into the development of the present conventional-view classifications. Nevertheless, the results presented so far in this book give a clear indication of some of the main features which such a classification might be expected to possess.

In the first place, as just noted, nothing of a properly empirical nature included in the present conventional-view classifications, would be excluded from a reverse-view classification. A reverse view includes, but is not limited to, the empirical elements in the conceptual structure of medicine. Indeed this is one area in which, as anticipated in chapter 3, disentangling fact from value (as in a reverse view) rather than suppressing value in favour of fact (as in the conventional view) could actually facilitate the progress of science in medicine. Certainly the conventional strategy for developing classifications of mental disorders, by following the empirical-scientific path beaten by physical medicine, is one which can have only limited success. In physical medicine, in which questions of value are usually not at issue diagnostically, this strategy can successfully be pursued essentially by ignoring such questions. But this is not the case in psychological medicine. In psychological medicine questions of value *are* sometimes at issue diagnostically (the criteria by which we evaluate mental-illness constituents not being widely settled or agreed, cf. chapter 5). Hence with a conventional-view approach to the classification of mental disorders, either these questions of value will be recognized for what they are and then excluded from the classifications, or they will not be so recognized and dealt with as though they were questions of fact. The former course has some utility, especially for (scientific) research. But for clinical work, to the extent that evaluative questions *are* raised by diagnosis in psychological medicine, the usefulness of our classifications can only be diminished by excluding them. In fact, though, it is the latter course, the course of treating questions of value as though they were questions of fact, which is perhaps the more common. But this course must founder altogether, according to the non-descriptivist conclusion of chapter 3, on the is–ought divide. At best, therefore, scientific research in this area will be wasted through misdirection, with science as it were knocking its head against an evaluative brick wall.

A first feature of a reverse-view classification would thus be clarification of its empirical elements. But with this feature goes a second – namely, clarification of its non-empirical elements. For with a reverse view, value, besides being disentangled from fact, is made fully explicit in its own right. Much of the analytical effort involved in developing the present reverse view was required in order to do just this, to bring to the surface and out into the open the evaluative element in the conceptual structure of medicine. Of course, merely to make explicit the evaluative element in the definitions in our classifications of mental disorders is not to resolve the difficulties with which this element is associated. But it is a first step. Instead of these difficulties being ignored or suppressed we are brought to face them, as it was put in chapter 3, full square. Then, at the very least, the more obvious confusions and contradictions among them can be avoided. Something of the need for this is apparent in the established classifications. In ICD-9, evaluation is not mentioned at all. In DSM-III, on the other hand, it is clearly there. It is there, for example, and centrally, in the very definition adopted of 'mental disorder'. This definition, although essentially in terms of 'disturbance of function', incorporates notions of distress and disability. Yet even here the element of evaluation is hardly more than implicit, the most explicitly evaluative term employed, "commendable", appearing only in a parenthetical part of the definition in which 'mental disorder' is marked off from 'social deviance' (DSM-III, p. 6). And it is presumably for this reason – it is because the evaluative element in this definition was not squarely in the sights of the editors of DSM-III – that in the body of the classification a number of mental disorders are actually defined contrary to the definition, in terms of social evaluative norms. Thus, the "essential feature" of conduct disorder is said to be a pattern of conduct "in which either the basic rights of others or major age-appropriate societal norms or rules are (seriously) violated" (DSM-III, p. 45). And the paraphilias, similarly, the "disorders" of sexual object choice (fetishism, sadism and so forth), are described as including those whose "only problem is the reaction of others to their behaviour" (DSM-III, p. 267).

The point here is not that DSM-III is in this respect less satisfactory than ICD-9 – indeed, in ICD-9 no definition of 'mental disorder' is attempted. The point is rather that if the evaluative element in both classifications (which, as an improvement on ICD-9, is at least perceptible in DSM-III) were made fully explicit, it could then be handled that much more effectively. And if this is true of evaluation generally, it comes out even more forcibly in respect of the particular *kind* of value which is expressed by 'illness', analysed, as it has been here, in terms of 'action failure'. For as we found in chapter 8, where evaluation generally is just perceptible in DSM-III, 'action', and the logical links between it and 'illness', surface repeatedly throughout both DSM-III and ICD-9. The basic logical distinction between illness and things that are done both to and by people, the positive and negative senses of ' "ordinary" doing' and each of the several components of 'action' (purposiveness, intentionality, voluntariness, control and so on) normally latent in ' "ordinary" doing', are all clearly visible as elements in the standard medical definitions of mental disorders. This relative visibility of 'action' compared with evaluation is only what we should expect from the results of chapter 7, since it is the particular kind of value which is expressed by 'illness', rather than evaluation as such, which is most often and most intractably problematic diagnostically (in the "mad versus bad" and similar issues as noted at the end of chapter 5). But if 'action' is visible in our classifications of mental disorders, it is not recognized squarely for what it is any more than evaluation is. Otherwise, how could 'anorexia nervosa' have come to be defined in ICD-9 essentially as "a persistent active refusal to eat" (p. 46), a definition which would include hunger strikers, for example? (There is of course more to the full syndrome than just this central symptom.) And how could 'encopresis' have come to be defined as "voluntary or involuntary" passage of stools, while 'enuresis' (without explanation or comment) is restricted to "involuntary" voiding of urine (ICD-9, p. 47)?

Similarly, in DSM-III, how could the expressions 'failure to resist' and 'unable to resist', despite their profoundly different implications (cf. chapter 8) have come to be used (apparently) as synonyms – for example, in defining the various "disorders of impulse control" (DSM-III, pp. 291–8)? With 'action', of course, perhaps even more so than with undifferentiated evaluation, making it explicit is only a first step towards resolving the conceptual difficulties with which it is associated. If this were not so, philosophers of action would have been out of business for some time now. But resolving these difficulties, at least in part, is necessary if the clarity and consistency of our definitions of mental disorders are to be improved. And recognizing the difficulties for what they are is at least a first step in this direction.

A reverse view thus has a number of important implications for the form which the definitions in our classifications of mental disorders should take. In a reverse-view classification the empirical elements in the definitions of individual disorders would be clarified, while the non-empirical elements – evaluation and the components of 'action' – would be made fully explicit. Non-empirical elements would not appear in the definition of *all* the disorders in such a classification, of course. As elements deriving from 'illness' rather than from 'disease', they would tend to appear in the definitions only of those disorders in respect of which (because indeed of the difficulties with which these elements are associated, cf. chapter 8) illness-diagnosis, instead of or as well as disease-diagnosis, is important clinically. But in the classification as a whole, these non-empirical elements would be there, and explicitly so.

Besides its implications for the definitions of individual disorders, however, a reverse view has implications for the overall structure of disease classifications. These implications are derived not from a reverse-view analysis of 'illness' as such but from the insights which can be derived from such an analysis into the similarities and differences between 'mental illness' and 'bodily illness'.

Consider first the similarities. Here the message of a reverse view is clear: namely, that in our present classifications, notwithstanding their development on the model of physical medicine, the parallels between mental and physical disorders are not likely to have been exploited fully. This is because the particular view of physical medicine on which they have been modelled, the conventional view is (according to a reverse view) itself a restricted view in which the full extent of these parallels has generally not been fully appreciated. This point was implicit in the comments made in chapter 5 about the conflation of 'illness' and 'disease' in much of the literature on the medical concepts. It comes out now, in relation to classification, explicitly, for example in the very limited use which is made in our present classifications of concepts such as 'wound' and 'disability'. The conventional view is dominated largely by the concept of 'disease'; therefore our present classifications of mental disorders have been developed largely as though they were classifications exclusively of diseases. Yet this is unduly restrictive, for even in physical medicine doctors are concerned with wounds and disabilities, as well as many other kinds of condition (cf. chapter 2). And in the ICD-9 itself, although many of its non-psychiatric sections are indeed made up of diseases, organized according to bodily parts and systems, two sections are given over to wounds and injuries, while many disabilities appear in a separate supplementary classification. But the psychiatric section of ICD-9 (section v), although actually called the mental *disorders* section, is developed as though it were just another section of diseases – diseases of the 'mental system', as it were, alongside diseases of the nervous system (section vi), diseases of the cardiovascular system (section vii) and so on. At the very least this has led to unnecessary tensions and difficulties in the development of the classification. The inclusion of certain stress-precipitated disorders, for example, was regarded by its authors as a "compromise" with their principle of symptomatic *disease* classification (ICD-9, p. 10), even though these disorders – induced psychoses (ICD-9, 298), acute reactions to stress (ICD-9, 308) and adjustment reactions (ICD-9, 309) – are in many important respects clear mental analogues of bodily trauma. But of greater importance, to the extent that such disorders – or at any rate our conceptions of them – are actually out there in the world, our classifications would be more useful clinically if the proper status of these disorders, as species of mental trauma, were made explicit. And in a reverse-view classification their status as species of mental trauma *would* be made explicit.

As with each of the foregoing features of a reverse-view classification, this of course raises questions for research. We need to be clearer, for example, about the differences between stress as defining 'mental trauma' and stress as defining HDf3-type (aetiologically based) diseases (cf. chapter 4). But such questions, from the point of view of diagnosis, are also clinically useful questions. Moreover, as for 'trauma', so also for 'disability'. Would it not be useful clinically – for example, in relation to medico-legal issues of responsibility – to explore the idea of 'psychopathy' not in the way that it has often been explored in recent literature, as a disease, but as a disability? After all, 'personality disorder', of which "sociopathic" or "amoral" personality disorder is a subcategory (ICD-9, 301.7), is defined as "continuing throughout most of adult life" (ICD-9, p. 38), a definition which implies, analogously with 'bodily disability' and in contrast to 'illness' and 'disease', little or no expectation of change (chapter 7).

However, if the similarities between physical medicine and psychological medicine have been obscured by the emphasis on 'disease' in the conventional view, so also – and perhaps to an even larger extent – have the differences. This is apparent, first, in the development of disease theory itself in psychological medicine. As already noted, the present symptomatically based classifications of mental disorders are conceived within a conventional view as merely preliminaries to the development of aetiologically based classifications similar to those which have been developed in physical medicine. And under a reverse view, too, there is no objection of principle to such a development, which, indeed, in so far as it is empirically sound, would be fully accommodated by it. However, under the conventional view, the *particular* disease theories which have developed in physical medicine – in terms of disturbances of function – are held, a priori even, to be paradigmatic (disturbances of function being held to mark out by definition what is from what is not illness, chapter 2). Whereas under a reverse view these particular disease theories occupy no such special place. In a reverse view, because 'illness' rather than 'disease' is held to be logically primary, the development of disease theory in medicine is recognized to be a posteriori, not a priori (chapter 4). And in a reverse view, therefore, while disease theory in psychological medicine *could* develop along the same lines as disease theory in physical medicine, there is no requirement, other than that of clinical utility, that it *should*. And while we may expect on general scientific grounds that disease theory in psychological medicine *will* develop, to some extent at any rate, along the same lines as disease theory in physical medicine – that is, to the extent that the brain sciences develop in the same way as the sciences of, say, the liver, lungs and heart have done – there are also grounds for expecting that in other respects it will *not*. This point is developed further in chapter 12. But what it comes down to is that the conceptual differences between the two kinds of medicine could well result in differences in the ways in which they develop scientifically. For example, the development of a dysfunction-based disease theory in physical medicine, as a clinically useful theory, has been made possible, *inter alia*, by bodily parts (and systems) and their functions being, if not clearly at least uncontentiously distinct from, respectively, persons and their actions (cf. chapter 3). Because of this there are no practically important conceptual barriers to thinking of our bodies as machines. But for mental parts and systems the corresponding distinctions are neither clear nor uncontentious. 'Mind' is conceptually more closely intertwined with 'person' than is 'body'; likewise 'mental function' is conceptually more closely intertwined with 'action' than 'bodily function' (chapter 6). And the latter distinctions, indeed, seem already to have been made in some respects more obscure by developments in the brain sciences. So for this reason alone, if for no others, the future development of disease theory in psychological medicine may be expected to diverge in some respects from, rather than to follow, disease theory in physical medicine.

Under a reverse view, then, although disease theory could develop in psychological medicine as it has in physical medicine, it is not obliged to. It is free to develop in its own way following developments in the brain sciences, and indeed in other relevant disciplines, philosophical or otherwise, to the extent that these are clinically useful in *psychological* medicine. It should be added, though, that for now, given the present state of the development of these disciplines, the largely symptomatic basis of disease theory in our classifications is as appropriate under a reverse view as it is under the conventional view. Hence it should not be expected that a reverse-view classification will look at present any different in this respect from conventional-view classifications. In both, diseases will be defined mainly symptomatically. In both, there will be the same nosological concerns; to establish reliable symptoms, to identify syndromes or other kinds of clinically useful groupings of these symptoms, to explore hierarchical and non-hierarchical arrangements of the groups identified, and so on. It is only in the future development of disease theory in psychological medicine that major differences between reverse- and conventional-view classifications can be expected to appear.

In respect of 'illness', however, in contrast to 'disease', the situation is quite different. Here there clearly would be differences, even now. Thus, we have seen already in this chapter that in the definitions of individual disorders the conceptual components of 'illness' – evaluation together with the several elements of 'action' – would be fully explicit in a reverse-view classification whereas they are by and large implicit, or at any rate not clearly recognized for what they are, in conventional-view classifications. This corresponds with the relative prominence in psychological medicine, as compared with physical medicine, of the concept of 'illness' (chapter 5). And this relative prominence would have to be reflected in the overall structure of a reverse-view classification. For once the components of 'illness' have been made fully explicit in the definitions of the individual disorders in the classification, "illness theory", reflecting the relationships between different kinds of illness, would have to be built into the structure of the classification, as well as disease theory.

Here, more than elsewhere, among reverse-view features now identified, much further research will be required before the shape which this illness theory should take can be settled, even provisionally. A reverse-view analysis of 'illness' provides a general theory within which this research could take place; and in so far as it is a coherent theory, it supplies a much-needed structural member even for our present classifications. It has indeed at least this much heuristic significance, that by analysing 'illness' *in terms of* 'action', it provides a single conceptual scheme within which the logical relationships between these otherwise apparently unconnected elements can be understood. But even so, and even if the reverse view developed here is right, there is much further work still to be done, both clinical and philosophical, before it can be readily translated into useful improvements in the structure of our classifications. Clinically, each, or a wide selection, of the definitions of the disorders in these classifications will have to be examined critically in the light of this reverse-view analysis. We made a tentative start on this with 'alcoholism' in chapter 8; and we will be looking in considerably more detail at 'psychosis' in chapter 10. But the next stage for such research, as emphasized in chapter 8, is to get back to real, raw clinical data. Then, philosophically, all the issues opened up by a reverse-view analysis must be considered: in particular, clarification of the elements of 'action', especially of the evaluative element in 'intention' (chapter 6); elucidation of the relationships between 'action' and 'function', and hence of that between 'illness' and 'disease' (chapter 7); and so on. The reverse-view analysis developed here has suggested certain lines along which philosophical research in these areas might be pursued (chapter 7). Moreover, as noted in chapter 8, such research is likely to be facilitated by the data derived from first-hand clinical investigation of a sufficiently wide range of mental disorders. But what all this amounts to is a lot of further work, clinical and philosophical, remaining to be done.

Still, for purposes of illustration, and setting caution aside, we might speculate on the future form of illness theory in a reverse-view classification as follows. In the conventional view, 'illness', in so far as it is distinguished from 'disease' at all, is thought of as a unitary concept – thus for Boorse, 'illness' means simply "serious disease" (chapter 3). But in a reverse view, 'illness', although a unitary concept to the extent that it is defined generally in terms of 'action failure', may take diverse forms – different kinds of illness being defined by different kinds of action failure, made up on the one hand of different kinds of illness constituent and on the other of different elements of 'action' (chapter 8). And one way to reflect this diversity of types of illness in the structure of our classifications would be by something akin to the periodic table in chemistry. In such a table, the columns could represent the main groups of constituents of illness (movements, sensations, affects, cognitions and so on), the rows its components (as elements of 'action'); then each cell, each intersection of row and column, would represent a particular kind of potential action failure – that is, a failure combining a particular kind of illness constituent with a particular element of action.

A table of this sort, if only as a framework for research, would be interestingly flexible in various ways. First, the particular rows and particular columns adopted could be changed according to the results of research (clinical and philosophical) into the structure of 'action'. Second, some of the cells, as potential kinds of action failure, might turn out not to correspond with any observed kind of illness, bodily or mental, and this would raise important questions for the research itself. Third, the kinds of illness actually observed might sometimes be found to correspond to more than one cell, either as composite illnesses (conflations of illnesses which in fact are distinct) or complex illnesses (illnesses defined by the combined failures of more than one element of 'action' and/or in respect of more than one constituent). In the latter case the observed groups of cells, not unlike the observed groups of chemical elements, might then reflect (and thus supply insights into) the structure of 'action' and hence of 'illness'. Fourth, disease theory would be automatically incorporated in the table; for, reflecting the logical priority of 'illness' over 'disease', diseases would be represented by whichever cells or groups of cells in the table correspond with those conditions which are *widely* regarded as illnesses, together with whatever families of disease concepts are, or already have been, derived from these conditions under the selective pressures of clinical utility (see chapter 4 generally, and chapter 7). So a reverse-view classification set out in this way would encompass, but not be limited to, the disease theories by which our present conventional-view classifications are largely shaped.

Thus, when illness theory is taken into account, a reverse-view classification would appear different in a number of respects from the present conventional-view classifications. It would contain the same empirical elements, but marked off more clearly from the non-empirical elements. And whereas disease theory within the classification would still be mainly symptomatically based, there would not be the same expectation that its future development be along the same lines as disease theory in physical medicine. Then again, the non-empirical elements – evaluation and the elements of 'action' – which are largely implicit in our present classifications would, where relevant, be fully explicit in the definitions of individual disorders. This would present additional requirements for research, over and above the existing requirement for scientific research into the empirical elements in these classifications. But it would at least allow a number of the confusions and contradictions in the definitions in our present classifications to be avoided. Furthermore, to the extent that these non-empirical elements are elements of 'illness', a reverse-view classification would reflect illness theory as well as disease theory in its overall structure, perhaps in a periodic table or such like. Finally, just as 'illness' as well as 'disease' would be made fully explicit in a reverse-view classification, so we should expect that the full range of medical concepts would be fully employed: besides (the predominant) 'illness' and 'disease', the concepts of 'wound' and 'disability' as described earlier, together with any others which may be relevant.

Diagnosis, the clinical process of deciding what is wrong with someone, would also look different within a reverse-view classification. Diagnosis in psychological medicine, like diagnosis in physical medicine, is essentially a two-stage process: the symptoms from which a person is suffering are first clarified by what is (presumed to be) an essentially empirical process, and they are then identified with one or more of the (presumed) diseases in the official classifications. This, at least, is the ideal. As noted earlier, in practice the identification of disease takes place within a wide range of individual variations on the official theme.

Within a reverse-view classification, however, diagnosis, although involving the same two stages of clarification and identification, would be at once more rigorous, more comprehensive and more apposite clinically. It would be more rigorous because in its first stage (of clarification) the empirical elements in diagnosis would be disentangled from the non-empirical: for example, description of a patient's condition would be disentangled from the value judgements involved in subsequently deciding whether, in virtue of that condition, the patient is ill – "condition-diagnosis" versus "illness-diagnosis" (cf. chapter 1). It would be more comprehensive because, in its second stage (of identification), the condition from which a patient is suffering would be identifiable within a range of concepts including but not limited to that of 'disease'; i.e., besides 'illness', such concepts as 'wound' and 'disability'. It would be more apposite clinically because, being both more rigorous and more comprehensive in the ways just described, it would be less procrustean. At any rate, there is a reasonable expectation that this would be so. For diagnosis in psychological medicine, as we have seen, regularly involves the concept of 'illness' (and other medical and non-medical concepts) as much as that of 'disease'. Moreover, in involving these concepts, diagnosis in psychological medicine, as we have also seen, regularly involves non-empirical as well as empirical issues. Hence there is a reasonable expectation that if diagnosis in psychological medicine is allowed to take place within a classification of "things wrong" in which these concepts and issues are fully represented, then the clinical facts should require less pushing and pulling and less stretching and squeezing than they do at present, in order to make them fit.

Whether, though, this turns out to be so, of course remains subject to the final test of actual clinical experience. And this test – and with it, therefore, substantive second outcome criterion support for a reverse-view analysis – is in turn dependent on the further detailed clinical and philosophical research which is necessary if a reverse-view classification is to become available for clinical use. Such a classification need not be complete, however, for it to be clinically useful. Indeed, if a reverse-view analysis *is* useful clinically, then historical precedent suggests that the various features of a reverse-view classification described here will emerge, piecemeal but progressively, in future revisions of the official classifications. This is simply a matter of survival of the fittest — that is, of the selective pressures of clinical utility continuing to operate in the future as they have in the past. For the (primary) usefulness of a reverse view is in respect of non-empirical clinical problems. But such problems are becoming increasingly important in medicine. Hence, if a reverse view *is* useful in dealing with problems of this kind, then it, or something like it, will inevitably become increasingly selected for in the future evolution of our classifications of mental disorders.

In fact, there are signs that this is already happening. In DSM-III, for example, as noted above, there is the appearance, for the first time explicitly in an official classification, of evaluation. Then again, there are a number of disorders in respect of which clinical research workers, although initially involved in straightforwardly empirical studies, have found themselves drawn to consider conceptual questions; asking, for example, precisely what is *meant* by 'bulimia nervosa' and seeking to explore this question by what amounts to an examination of ordinary medical usage (i.e., by a detailed examination of the criteria adopted in making the diagnosis in actual clinical practice; Fairburn, 1988). And questions of meaning have of course always been important in relation to medico-legal and ethical issues (chapter 1). Then again, there is the recent shift, noted earlier in this chapter, in the basis of our classifications from aetiology to symptomatology (with ICD-8). Conventionally this shift has been regarded, as indeed it was described above, as a shift *back* to an earlier "Sydenham-type" stage in the development of disease theory, preparatory to the emergence of aetiological theories similar to those which have appeared in physical medicine. In a reverse view of the medical concepts, however, this shift is seen to be a shift not merely from one kind of disease theory to another, but *towards* illness. For it is a shift up along the logical chain described in chapter 4, from HDf2 (aetiologically-based) diseases, to HDf1 (symptomatically based) diseases. And this chain leads on through HDv ('disease' used as a value term) to the subcategory Id (of conditions widely regarded as illnesses) and thus to 'illness' itself – that is, to the category, I, of conditions which may be regarded as illnesses, those conditions which, collectively, would be represented in the hypothetical periodic table described a moment ago.

So the signs of an emerging reverse-view classification are already there. And the potential contribution of the present analysis towards improved diagnosis and classification in psychological medicine can thus be seen as more facilitatory than innovatory. This analysis, if right, allows these signs to be recognized for what they are, and it thus gives structure and direction to the underlying trends in classification which they represent. Equally, however, to the extent that classification in medicine is now, as historically it has always been, needdriven, the appearance of these signs at this time provides good second outcome criterion evidence in support of it.

10
Treatment

As with diagnosis, so with treatment, a reverse-view analysis is relevant more to the non-empirical than to the empirical problems of clinical practice. However, where in the case of diagnosis its relevance to these problems is direct, in the case of treatment its relevance is mainly indirect. This is because in the case of diagnosis the conceptual problems in respect of which a reverse view is particularly relevant are overt, whereas in the case of treatment such problems are mostly hidden within problems which, outwardly, are ethical, medico-legal or political in nature. In this chapter the relevance of a reverse view to problems of this kind will be illustrated by considering compulsory psychiatric treatment. Such treatment is subject to strong but conflicting moral intuitions. It thus raises a number of important ethical, medico-legal and political issues. However, clarification of these issues is in part dependent on clarification of the concept of mental illness − hence the contribution of our reverse-view analysis, which, as we will see, both increases understanding and supplies a framework for future research in this area.

The argument is developed in two main stages. In the first half of the chapter, three conceptual fences are found in the way of clarification of the grounds of compulsory treatment, fences raised respectively by the concepts of 'mental illness', of 'psychotic mental illness' and of 'delusion'. The conventional view of the logical structure of medicine is shown to fail at each of these fences, in the sense that it gives results which are inconsistent with the intuitions, both ethical and clinical, of everyday medical practice. This failure of the conventional view then leads, in the second half of the chapter, to a reverse-view account consistent with, and thus clarifying, these intuitions.

The clinical context of compulsory psychiatric treatment is illustrated by the following case history. Mr A.B., a 48-year-old bank manager, came with his wife to the casualty department of his local hospital. He complained of burning pains in his face and head. While he was waiting to be seen, his general practitioner telephoned the casualty officer. She told him that she had persuaded Mr A.B. to attend casualty not so much because of his burning pains but because she thought he was seriously depressed. Over the last three to four weeks he had become gloomy and preoccupied and had lost interest in his work. His sleep had been disturbed – he had been waking earlier than usual – and he had lost weight. Normally he was a hard-working, cheerful extrovert. However, he had had periods of depression before, and during the last of these (when he had complained similarly of head and facial pains) he had made a sudden and nearly fatal suicide attempt. Mr A.B. had become angry at his general practitioner's suggestion that he see a psychiatrist but had agreed to come to casualty for further investigation of his head pains.

The casualty officer found Mr A.B. to be morose and unsmiling. He gave a clear and consistent description of his pains but was guarded and suspicious when asked about his health generally. Questioned directly about previous illnesses, he became frankly irritated, telling the casualty officer to get on with whatever tests his general practitioner wanted done. The casualty officer then talked to Mr A.B.'s wife, who confirmed the recent changes in his mood and said that he was behaving very much as he had before his suicide attempt. The duty psychiatrist was then called. In the course of a careful physical and neurological examination he was able to question Mr A.B. further about his health. Mr A.B. now admitted that he believed he had "advanced brain cancer". However, at the suggestion that he stay in hospital, he again became angry, saying that there was "no point any more", and that all he needed was "something for the pain". The psychiatrist explained that he had found no signs whatsoever of brain cancer, and that he thought in fact Mr A.B. had become depressed again. He said that further tests were needed – skull X-ray, electroencephelogram and so on – but that the burning pains were almost certainly due to depression. Mr A.B., however, refused even to consider this possibility, saying that brain cancer did not always "show itself", and that anyone with brain cancer would be likely to feel as he had been feeling.

At this stage the psychiatrist decided that in view of the high suicide risk, Mr A.B.'s protestations notwithstanding, he had no option but to consider compulsory treatment under the Mental Health Act 1983. In his view, as required by the Act, Mr A.B. was suffering from a mental illness, which, in the interests of his own safety, warranted detention in hospital for further assessment and treatment. He discussed this with Mr A.B.'s wife and with his general practitioner, both of whom agreed. A Section-2 order was accordingly made, and Mr A.B. was admitted to the psychiatric ward. There, on antidepressant drug therapy, he made a full recovery over the next eight weeks. At his first outpatient follow-up he admitted to the psychiatrist that he had agreed to attend casualty originally only because he thought he would be given something stronger than aspirin for his pains, and that he had been planning to use this to kill himself. Now, far from wanting to kill himself, he was concerned about the risks of a further relapse. In addition to routine follow-up, therefore, which would continue for some time, he agreed that he or his wife should contact either his general practitioner or the psychiatrist immediately if his head pains or gloomy mood returned.

This case, which is a clinically standard one, shows just how compelling is the moral intuition under which most compulsory treatment is carried out. Although it involves a clear infringement of liberty, few would disagree with the psychiatrist that he had "no option" but to proceed as he did. Indeed, he might well have been judged negligent had he not done so. This moral intuition, furthermore, is one which is shared worldwide, legislation similar to the United Kingdom's Mental Health Act 1983 existing in many other countries (McGarry and Chodoff, 1981). Nor is it merely a modern intuition. In the nineteenth century, for example, no less an advocate of individual freedom than John Stuart Mill, in his treatise *On Liberty*, excluded by implication the mentally ill from his libertarian guiding principle.

Yet, widely shared as this intuition may be, compulsory treatment, even in a clinically standard case like Mr A.B.'s, has its opponents. Some have argued that the erosion of liberty involved is simply too high a price to pay for the benefits which such treatment may bring in individual cases (Szasz, 1963). Others, more radical, have seen in it a conspiracy: Foucault, for example, who is among those who deny the reality of mental illness, has claimed that all compulsory "treatment", so called, is really a form of political coercion (1973). We may dismiss such claims. We may, with Wing (1978, p. 244), regard as "repellent" the attitude of those who would refuse compulsory treatment even to a suicidally depressed patient like Mr A.B. But even so, the possibility, at least, must be admitted that in some countries, in Russia for example, compulsory psychiatric treatment may actually have been used in the way that Foucault describes, as a means of political control (Bloch, 1981). It is true that this is usually denied by the doctors concerned. But the issues raised by such denials serve only to underline the extent to which compulsory treatment is open if not to (deliberate) abuse then to (inadvertent) misuse. After all, not all clinical cases are as straightforward as Mr A.B.'s. And it is public concern about the risks of both abuse and misuse of compulsory treatment which lies behind the protective clauses built into the Mental Health Act 1983, and into other similar legislation around the world. Decisions about compulsory treatment, although essentially medical decisions, and life-and-death decisions at that, are none the less firmly among those which society is unwilling to leave solely to doctors alone (cf. ch. 1). In Mr A.B.'s case, for instance, the Section-2 order not only required a second opinion (provided by the general practitioner), but it could not have been made at all other than on the application of Mr A.B.'s wife (as his nearest relative) or on that of a non-medical "approved" social worker (that is, one authorized under the act). Furthermore, after fourteen days, either Mr A.B. or his wife or an approved social worker could have applied to a predominantly non-medical Mental Health Review Tribunal for the order to be rescinded.

Compulsory treatment, then, on the one hand morally imperative, is on the other subject to moral doubts and difficulties. The standard intuition is that such treatment, at least in a case like Mr A.B.'s, is not only justified but positively required in order to satisfy a doctor's obligations to his patient. Yet compulsory treatment is opposed altogether by some, abused (apparently) by others, and so uncertain in application as to require multiple safeguards against its misuse. And there the matter could rest. Indeed, as Wing found (1978, ch. 6), so powerful are the passions raised by the conflicting moral intuitions to which compulsory treatment is subject that it can be hazardous to proceed further. Yet here, surely, if anywhere in medical ethics, there is a clear need to move forward, as Hare puts it (1981b), from level-1 to level-2 moral thinking; from the level of direct moral intuitions, essential in the day-to-day conduct of our lives, to a level of critical reflection on the principles embodied in these intuitions. For in clarifying the principle under which compulsory treatment is (intuitively) justified, we may hope to meet more decisively the arguments of the opponents of such treatment, to deal more effectively with cases of abuse and to reduce in everyday clinical work the risks of misuse.

And at first, in moving forward from level-1 to level-2 moral thinking, all goes well. For the principle under which compulsory treatment is justified turns out, straightforwardly, to be none other than the Hippocratic principle. Thus, according to this principle, a doctor's decisions about the treatment of a patient should in general be governed by the interests of that patient. Normally, the best guide to a patient's interest is what the patient, having been informed appropriately, actually wants. Yet this is not always so. Hence, where it is not, compulsory treatment, treatment which the patient does not actually want, may be required to satisfy the doctor's obligations to that patient under the Hippocratic principle. In the literature, Glover (1970), Wing (1978) and others have illustrated this point variously with such uncontentious cases as children, mental defectives, the dementing and the confused.

But now comes a difficulty, for, as Flew (1973) has emphasized, what is morally problematic about compulsory psychiatric treatment is not the principle as such, nor its application to the uncontentious cases just mentioned, but its application, as in Mr A.B.'s case, specifically to mental illness. Certainly, there is *something* about mental illness in virtue of which it seems (to many) to fall intuitively within the principle of compulsory treatment. This is the standard intuition, so firmly and so widely held. But this something is something specific to mental illness. Mr A.B., indeed, whose case is clinically standard remember, stands in direct contrast to the uncontentious cases cited above in being an adult patient who is fully conscious and of normal intelligence. Furthermore, in respect of this "something", mental illness is different not only from other kinds of mental disorder but also from any kind of physical disorder. Some physical disorders, it is true, can be treated against the patient's wishes in the interests of others (for example, if the patient is a typhoid carrier). And in the United Kingdom, at least, there are various so-called "care" provisions which can occasionally be used (mainly for elderly patients) with physical disorders (Muir Gray, 1985). But there is no Physical Health Act corresponding to the Mental Health Act 1983, for there are no physical illnesses, as there are mental illnesses, in respect of which the compulsory treatment of a fully conscious adult patient of normal intelligence would be justified, not for the protection of others (though there is provision also for this in the Mental Health Act 1983), but, as with Mr A.B. in the interests of the patient's own health or safety. (Though compulsory treatment of a physical illness may possibly be justified where refusal of treatment arises from a mental illness.)

Here, then, is a first conceptual fence – a fence raised by the concept of 'mental illness' – in the way of clarification of the principle under which compulsory treatment in a case like Mr A.B.'s is justified. The standard ethical intuition is that compulsory treatment of this kind is justified only for *mental* illness. Clarification of the principle underlying this intuition thus involves providing some explanation for why this should be so. Why just mental illness? Why not physical illness also?

And even at this first fence the conventional view stumbles. It stumbles, first, because with respect to the standard intuition about compulsory treatment it looks, as it were, the wrong way. Thus, if the standard intuition is right, what needs to be clarified is what there is about mental illness which makes it *different* from physical illness. But the conventional view – at any rate as promoted by the supporters of 'mental illness' – is concerned rather with the *similarities* between them (chapter 1). However, a second, more serious reason for the stumbling of the conventional view at this fence is that it leads to conclusions which are actually inconsistent with the standard intuition. Thus, although there are important general ethical issues involved here (cf. Macklin, 1982), the justification of compulsory psychiatric treatment, as a specifically *medical* intervention, is dependent on the validity of the concept of mental illness – if Mr A.B. had not really been ill, there might have been, say, religious or humanitarian or paternalistic grounds for preventing him from committing suicide, but there would not have been the specifically Hippocratic grounds required to justify the use of specifically medical treatment – let alone compulsory medical treatment – to this end. However, according to the conventional view, the validity of the concept of 'mental illness' depends on its similarity to the concept of 'physical illness', for 'physical illness' is the paradigm and 'mental illness' is to be measured against it (chapter 1). And 'physical illness', according to the standard intuition, is quite different in this respect from 'mental illness'. Hence, granted the dependence of the justification of compulsory treatment on the validity of 'mental illness', this is inherently incompatible with the standard ethical intuition restricting such treatment to the mentally ill.

This is equally true for the supporter and the opponent of compulsory treatment. For the supporter, the implication of the conventional view (that 'physical illness' is the paradigm) has to be that the standard ethical intuition is, if not wrong, at least misdirected. Thus, if 'physical illness' is the paradigm, then, contrary to the standard intuition, it should be physical illness, not mental illness, in respect of which compulsory treatment is the more readily justified. Or at any rate, though still contrary to the standard intuition, compulsory treatment should be no less readily justified in respect of physical illness than mental. (This latter conclusion is indeed that to which Glover (1970) is in effect drawn.) For the opponent of compulsory treatment, on the other hand, the implication of the conventional view is that if compulsory treatment is not justified for physical illnesses as the standard intuition implies, then, 'physical illness' being the paradigm, neither is it justified for mental illnesses. The opponent, indeed, could combine the conventional view with the fact that the standard intuition differentiates in this way between mental illness and physical illness, to provide a demonstration that compulsory treatment of the mentally ill is not justified. For he could argue that this differentiation points to there being at least *some* difference between 'mental illness' and 'physical illness'. This difference has then to be either logically trivial or logically essential. If it is trivial, then the concept of 'mental illness' stands – because it satisfies the paradigm 'physical illness' – but compulsory treatment falls – because it springs from some feature of mental illness which on the conventional view is incidental to its status as illness. But if the difference is logically essential, then 'mental illness' itself falls – because it is essentially different from 'physical illness' – and compulsory treatment falls with it.

The conventional view, however, if stumbling at this first fence, actually refuses at the second. The second fence in the way of clarification of the grounds of compulsory treatment is raised by the fact that some mental illnesses, specifically psychotic mental illnesses, are more likely than others to be treated compulsorily. Under the Mental Health Act 1983 any mental illness can in principle be treated compulsorily. In practice, however, such treatment is very largely confined to psychotic illnesses – Mr A.B. had a psychotic illness, an "affective psychosis" (ICD-9) or "major affective disorder with psychotic features" (DSM-III).

Now, as a matter of level-1 moral thinking, thinking at the intuitive level, there is no mystery here. For in at least three respects psychotic mental illnesses are paradigm mental illnesses: compared with non-psychotic illnesses, they are more reliably identifiable (that is, there is a good degree of agreement between observers in their identification clinically, Wing *et al.*, 1974); they compare favourably with physical illnesses in the extent to which they are ordinarily thought of as diseases (Campbell *et al.* 1979); and, corresponding as they do to the traditional 'insane', they have been thought of as diseases at

least back to classical times (Kenny, 1969). Hence, if it is right –
as it is standardly taken to be right – that compulsory treatment
of fully conscious adult patients of normal intelligence should
be confined to *mental* illnesses, then it is right – as it is standardly
taken to be right – that such treatment be further confined
largely to the paradigmatic *psychotic* mental illnesses. Indeed,
the fact that the standard intuition is consistent in this respect is
an important level-1 endorsement of it. However, for level-2
moral thinking, rather more is required. For level-2 moral
thinking, explanation is required. Hence, just as at the first
fence the question had to be raised "why mental illness?", so
here, at the second, the question has to be raised "why
psychotic mental illness?" But the conventional view, far from
addressing this question, fails to give any account at all of the
very distinction between psychotic and non-psychotic mental
illness. And the reaction of the proponents of the conventional
view to this failure has been, not self-doubt, but doubt about,
and hence a tendency to reject, the distinction itself.

In its essentials, the conventional argument runs thus. It starts
with the clinical observation that psychotics (characteristically)
lack what is called "insight" (ICD-9, p. 21) or "reality testing"
(DSM-III, p. 367). But what does this mean? Does it mean that
they are irrational? For certainly psychotics are irrational. But
then so is everyone else at times. Hence 'psychosis' – at least if it
is to justify compulsory psychiatric treatment – must mean a
particular kind of irrationality, amounting to irrationality *as*
illness. Severe irrationality then? For certainly psychotics are
severely irrational. But then in what sense "severe"? For there
are non-psychotic mental illnesses no less harmful (Glover's
illness criterion, 1970), no less incapacitating (Flew's criterion,
1973), and no less distressing and disabling (Wing's criterion,
1978). Furthermore, the difference between psychotic and non-
psychotic patients is more qualitative than quantitative, in that,
roughly, whereas non-psychotic patients (characteristically)
recognize that they are mentally ill, psychotic patients (characteristically) do not: this is the particular "insight" they lack, this
is the particular "reality" they fail to test – witness Mr A.B.,
who thought he had brain cancer when everyone else thought
he was suffering from depression.

The psychotic's particular irrationality, then, has to do with getting his diagnosis wrong. But the conventional view of diagnosis, as we saw in the last chapter, is that it is essentially a matter of fact. On this view it has to do with data, with evidence, with knowledge; with what Aubrey Lewis (1934) described as the "correct perception" of signs and symptoms. On this view, therefore, as Aubrey Lewis pointed out, the insight which the psychotic patient is said to lack turns out to be the same not only as that which some non-psychotic mentally ill patients lack but also as that which some physically ill patients lack. Aubrey Lewis cited a doctor with acromegaly who for twenty years failed to perceive his own progressive facial disfigurement despite the evidence before his eyes every morning when he shaved; and a boy with optic atrophy who believed firmly, and despite contrary test results, not only that he could still see with his blind eye, but that the vision in that eye was improving. Both patients, in Aubrey Lewis's view, lacked "insight". Both failed to "test reality". All in all, therefore, the harder the psychotic versus non-psychotic distinction is pressed, the more, on the conventional view, it appears to be a distinction without a difference. And on this view one is thus forced to conclude, as Aubrey Lewis concluded, that it is an invalid distinction and one which, having lost whatever usefulness it may once have had, should now be abandoned.

This conclusion, with Aubrey Lewis in 1934, could well have been right. And, influential as Aubrey Lewis has been in psychiatry, it is a conclusion which many coming after him have thought to be right. Indeed the academic fashion nowadays is, if not wholly to reject the distinction between psychotic and non-psychotic mental illnesses, at least to distance oneself from it. The authors of ICD-9, for example, while retaining psychosis as a major category of mental disorder, apologize for it as a "working compromise" (ICD-9, p. 11) necessary "in view of its wide use" (ICD-9, p. 35). And in DSM-III it disappears altogether as a separate category of mental disorder. Yet the fact of the matter, as the ICD-9 authors themselves acknowledge, is that the distinction persists. Fifty years on from Aubrey Lewis, and despite, as it were, our best efforts at suppression, it persists. It persists in ordinary medical usage, with terms like "antipsychotic drug", "puerperal psychosis" and "psychotic symptom" continuing to be used as freely as ever, and in academic journals, subject to editorial scrutiny, as much as in everyday informal clinical discourse. And it persists, too, in our classifications: in ICD-9 explicitly; but even in DSM-III implicitly, in the continued use in that classification of the adjective 'psychotic' and, clearest sign of all, in the retention of a category "psychotic disorders not elsewhere classified" (DSM-III, pp. 199–203).

But if the distinction between psychotic and non-psychotic mental illness persists, then, according to the "survival of the fittest" argument of the last chapter, this is itself good *prima-facie* evidence that, contrary to Aubrey Lewis's conclusion, it really does mark something important. Given that it is used, and goes on being used, then it is likely that it is useful – which, of course, in respect of compulsory psychiatric treatment at least, the standard intuition itself would suggest that it is. Since such treatment is (intuitively) confined largely to psychotic illnesses, the distinction, it would (intuitively) seem, really does mark a clinically important difference; and a difference, furthermore, not only from non-psychotic mental illnesses, but also from all physical illnesses. For (standing Aubrey Lewis's examples on their heads) the insight which may be lacking in cases of physical illness (as cited by Aubrey Lewis), in whatever other ways it may be similar to the psychotic's lack of insight, differs from it crucially in that (intuitively) it is *not* taken to justify compulsory treatment. And this remains true even for cases of physical illness more seriously and more immediately life-threatening, through lack of insight, than those described by Aubrey Lewis. Suppose, for example, that Mr A.B. had been like another patient, Mr C.D., who really did have brain cancer but who refused – as patients with so serious a condition sometimes do refuse – to believe the diagnosis. In that case, compulsory treatment, drug treatment or radiotherapy without his consent, far from being ethically justified would have constituted a legal assault. Of course, it is open to the Aubrey Lewis school to argue that the intuitively perceived difference here, between psychotic and non-psychotic failures of insight –

the one justifying, the other not justifying compulsory treatment – is illusory. But this leads to inconsistencies similar to
those thrown up by the conventional view at fence 1 – namely,
inconsistencies with the standard intuition. For if it were true,
then either all mental illnesses, psychotic and non-psychotic
alike, should be equally subject to compulsory treatment or
none should be – alternatives, therefore, in equal and opposite
ways at variance with the standard intuitive restriction of
compulsory treatment largely to psychotic illnesses.

For the conventional view there is thus something of a
conflict here. There is a wish to give up the psychotic versus
non-psychotic distinction, yet an inability to do without it.
Which brings us to our third conceptual fence, that raised by
the concept of 'delusion'. For this conflict has resulted in the
development of a conceptual split – a sort of logical double
think – through which, in effect, while the general concept of
'psychosis' is rejected, particular psychotic symptoms, of which
delusions are the most important, are retained. Noun and
adjective, for example, are split. The noun 'psychosis' is out, it
is considered too ill-defined for respectable use in medicine,
while the adjective 'psychotic' – denoting conditions in which
delusions and other psychotic symptoms characteristically occur – is in. This, as just noted, is the drift of DSM-III, which,
apparently, ICD-10 is set to follow (Sartorius, 1988). Similarly,
classification and clinical use are split. In the recent *Oxford
textbook of psychiatry*, for example, Gelder, Gath and Mayou
(1983, p. 71) argue that for purposes of classification the term
psychosis embraces so wide a range of conditions "... there is
little to be gained in bringing them together". Hence "the
diagnostic category of psychosis is of little value in clinical
practice". But in the following paragraph they say that for
"everyday clinical use ... the term psychosis ... is a convenient
collective term ... useful for communication". What it collects
is not specified here as such. However, three definitions of
'psychosis' are implied in the book (one on p. 70, two on p. 71);
each of these is symptomatically based; and of the symptoms
given, only hallucinations and delusions are common to all
three (as indeed they are to the various DSM-III lists of
psychotic symptoms, DSM-III, pp. 202–3, 367–8). Further-

more, of these two symptoms delusions are in an important sense phenomenologically basic, since true hallucinations are distinguished from pseudohallucinations (in one sense of this term) by the presence of what amounts to a delusional belief in the reality of the hallucinatory perception (see Taylor, 1981. The phenomenology of all these symptoms is described in more detail later on.)

The reason for this splitting is not hard to see. From the conventional point of view delusions offer all the advantages of the psychoses generally, apparently without any of the disadvantages. Like psychoses generally, delusions can be identified reliably (Wing *et al.*, 1974); they are ordinarily thought of as symptoms of illness (being central to the phenomenology for example of schizophrenia in Campbell *et al.*'s 1979 study of conditions ordinarily thought of as diseases); and they are closely associated with the historical notion of insanity (Jaspers, 1913b). Also, delusions, more so than other symptoms, involve lack of insight – "*ex hypothesi*" even (as Aubrey Lewis put it in his 1934 paper). And this ties in with the fact that just as most mentally ill patients who are treated compulsorily are psychotic, so they are deluded – Mr A.B. was deluded.

Delusions, however, in contrast to the psychoses generally, are, in the conventional view, readily definable. In Harré and Lamb's *Dictionary of physiological and clinical psychology* (1986), for example, 'psychosis' is, I believe, the only term in the whole dictionary for which no initial summary definition is given. 'Delusion', on the other hand, is defined, straightforwardly and without qualification, as "a false belief, held despite evidence to the contrary, and one which is not explicable in terms of the patient's educational and cultural background. It is held with complete conviction and cannot be shaken by argument." Essentially the same definition is found in most modern textbooks of psychiatry and psychology. And the definition is, indeed, highly satisfactory from the conventional point of view. It is descriptively based, none of its elements entailing a value judgement. And it is eminently capable of assimilation to the conventional analysis of 'disease' in terms of 'dysfunction' – delusions, being held with conviction despite evidence and/or arguments to the contrary and being culturally atypical, suggest impaired reasoning abilities, which, effacing any difficulties of epistemological relativism, issue in beliefs which are, in fact, false. Flew, for example, makes this explicit (1973, Part 1.16). And he goes on to argue, as many others have done (for example, Glover, 1970), first, that it is on this implied defect of reason that the justification of compulsory treatment in a case like Mr A.B.'s rests; and second, that the criterion of falsity, as the hallmark of a delusional belief, provides the one sure defence against the abuse and misuse of such treatment.

QED, then, at this third fence for the conventional view? 'Delusion', unlike the wider term 'psychosis', proving to be readily definable, and in terms not merely consistent with the conventional view but (and thereby) fully substantiating the standard intuitive moral grounds of compulsory treatment of (at least deluded) mentally ill patients? Closer inspection, however, shows, on the contrary, that at this third fence the conventional view, having stumbled at the first, and refused at the second, now finally falls. It falls, first, because, contrary to the conventional view, the conventional definition of 'delusion' does *not* in fact substantiate the intuitive moral grounds of compulsory treatment. Certainly there is nothing in the definition as it stands – that is, without the addition of the conventionally implied defect of reason – that would supply the logical element of pathology necessary to the specifically Hippocratic grounds required for compulsory treatment. Thus, delusions may indeed be, as the definition says, culturally atypical beliefs "not explicable in terms of the patient's educational and cultural background". But there is nothing in itself pathological about that. To suggest otherwise is to invite the worst excesses of paternalistic totalitarianism. Similarly, delusions may indeed be incorrigible beliefs "held with conviction despite evidence and/or arguments to the contrary". But there is nothing pathological about that either. Mere conviction is not a mark of pathology. And with *any* disputed belief, not just with a delusional belief, there must be someone for whom the evidence and/or arguments are *not* "to the contrary". Nor is consensus a sufficient guide. Consensus is relied on conventionally – for example, by Aubrey Lewis (1934) and in DSM–III (p. 356). But consensus proscribes, besides delusions, all that "intellectual individualism" which Einstein, no less, regarded as inseparable from innovation (Einstein, quoted in Maher and Ross, 1984). All in all, then, a false belief (like a delusion), even though (like a delusion) incorrigible, even though (like a delusion) culturally atypical, is, in the absence of defect of reason, no more than a mistaken belief. And simple mistake, though possibly supplying other grounds for interfering with what someone wants, does not supply the required Hippocratic grounds. This, by the way, of course remains true even though, as in Mr A.B.'s case, the subject subsequently, post-treatment as it were, acquiesces in the view that his original belief was mistaken. Shades here of George Orwell's "1984" Ministry of Truth!

But even with the addition of the conventionally implied defect of reason, the conventional definition still does not substantiate the intuitive grounds of compulsory treatment. For the defect conventionally implied is no more than the same cognitive defect implied by the conventional (Aubrey-Lewis-style) analysis of 'lack of insight'; it has to do with erroneous interpretation of evidence, with false argument and so on. This is consistent, at least, since lack of insight is the main clinical marker of psychosis, and delusion is the main psychotic symptom (though rejection of the former alongside acceptance of the latter requires the logical double-think described a moment ago). However, the difficulty for the conventional view is that as noted earlier, cognitive defects of this or similar kinds, though perfectly sound species of pathology, already supply the Hippocratic grounds for compulsory treatment in cases of mental deficiency and of dementia. No harm in this of course, so far as it goes. But in making cognitive defect the grounds of compulsory treatment also in cases of mental illness, the conventional view implies the assimilation of mental illness – in respect of the grounds of compulsory treatment – to mental deficiency and dementia. Which is counter-intuitive. Intuitively, as has been noted, the grounds of compulsory treatment in a (clinically standard) case of mental illness like that of Mr A.B., are quite different from those in cases of mental deficiency or dementia. And anyway, if it were as simple as that, why should compulsory treatment of the mentally ill be contentious in ways and to an extent that compulsory treatment of the mentally defective and the demented is not? Thus, to the counter-intuitive implications of the conventional view of 'mental illness' at the first and second fences have now to be added counter-intuitive implications at the third. Increasingly, therefore, it seems that in respect of compulsory psychiatric treatment, either the conventional view or the standard intuition must go.

Preferring therefore as we do, the primary data represented by the standard intuition, it comes as no surprise to find that the conventional definition of 'delusion' is in fact in all material respects, wrong. This is the second reason for the fall of the conventional view at this third fence. It is also the decisive reason, since the conventional definition is wrong for that most decisive of reasons, inconsistency with the clinical facts. In the first place, there is simply no evidence for the cognitive defect which is conventionally implied. Even with (clinically) unequivocal delusions, there is usually no defect of logical thinking as such (Maher and Ross, 1984). Indeed, cognitive defect, when present, is an ancillary symptom, contributing more to the differentiation of one psychotic condition from another than to the definition of psychotic disorders as a group. Thus, memory impairment is among the features marking out the organic psychoses (ICD-9, p. 21); and loosening of the associative links between thoughts is a feature of schizophrenia (ICD-9, p. 26). These ancillary symptoms, furthermore, when present, far from contributing to the development of delusions, actually interfere, if not with their inception, at least with their elaboration – just as, of course, they interfere with the elaboration of normal beliefs and ideas. In particular, delusions in an organic psychosis (for example, a dementia) are, like normal beliefs in this condition, of poor quality – minimally elaborated, only transiently sustained and emotionally shallow. Other ancillary symptoms, it is true, may have other more subtle cognitive effects. Marked mood change, for example, elevated in hypomanic disorders or depressed in depressive disorders, may act as a cognitive filter, influencing the selection and assessment of evidence (Teasedale et al., 1980). And this in turn may influence the content of delusional (as it does that of non-delusional) thinking – Mr A.B.'s hypochondriacal delusion that he had brain cancer was a typical depressive delusion. But the best quality delusions of all, complex and wide ranging in content, held with conviction over many years and of deep personal significance, occur in the paranoid psychoses (ICD-9, p. 31), psychotic conditions in which there are generally no ancillary symptoms at all. Indeed, in such conditions, the more intelligent the patient, the more cognitively competent he or she is, the better will be the quality of the delusions – as in Maher and Ross's case of a postgraduate physicist, the salient features of whose delusions occupy four pages of close-set type (Maher and Ross, 1987, pp. 385–8).

Of course, the conventional reply to all this has to be that while no generalized cognitive defect is necessarily associated with delusions, the features of delusions themselves, those by which they are conventionally defined – their falsity, incorrigibility and cultural atypicality – all point to at least a restricted defect. However, the plain fact of clinical life is that, notwithstanding the wide acceptance of the conventional definition, not all delusions show all or even any of these features. Many beliefs identified clinically as delusions are indeed false and/or incorrigible and/or culturally atypical. But not all. Certainly not all delusions are culturally atypical. Mr A.B.'s wasn't. His belief that he had brain cancer was a belief fully consistent with the educational and cultural background of a 48-year-old English bank manager. In any case, we distinguish, as do people even in less sophisticated cultures, delusional from non-delusional varieties of beliefs with the same general content (see, for example, Risso and Boker's account of delusions of witchcraft, 1968).

Then again, not all delusions are, as the conventional definition requires, incorrigible. They are held with conviction, certainly. But the evidence and/or arguments said (conventionally) to be "contrary" to them are often ambiguous or lacking altogether. This was true of Maher and Ross's postgraduate physicist. It was also true to some extent of Mr A.B. Mr A.B.'s belief was incorrigible in the sense that he was so convinced he had brain cancer that he was unwilling to consider that he might simply be depressed. But as to the evidence and/or arguments for and against this, his symptoms indeed could, as he claimed, have been due to brain cancer. Sometimes depression *is* due to brain cancer; and the lesion, if small and deeply placed, *can*, as Mr A.B. argued, escape detection, even with sophisticated tests. This is unlikely but far from impossible. Such cases have actually been reported (Lishman, 1978, Ch. 6). Thus, while Mr A.B. may have got the odds wrong (Hemsley and Garety, 1986), this amounts at most to a quantitative deviation from the biases which are a feature of normal belief formation (Rachman, 1983). Mr A.B.'s belief, contrary to Flew's criterion for true delusions, was not "wholly indefensible" (Flew, 1973, p. 94); nor, contrary to Glover's criterion, was the evidence against it "overwhelming" (Glover, 1970, pp. 134–5). And Mr A.B.'s case, you will recall, was not marginal. It was a clinically standard case which called unequivocally (according to the standard intuition) for compulsory treatment. In the event, it is true, Mr A.B.'s belief that he had brain cancer did turn out to be wrong. It thus satisfied at least one of the three elements of the conventional definition, the element indeed which as noted earlier, Flew sees as providing the only sure defence against improper use of compulsory treatment. But as to that, delusional beliefs, though commonly false, often bizarrely so, are, perhaps surprisingly, sometimes not false at all.

This last observation – that delusions are not always false beliefs – constitutes a conceptual watershed or divide between the conventional and a reverse view. On the one hand it provides final proof of the inadequacy of the conventional definition of 'delusion', a definition correctly describing many delusions but failing to catch the essence. On the other hand, it is the key to a reverse-view formulation of 'delusion' which, extended to 'psychotic mental illness' and then to 'mental illness', will enable us to get back over each of the three (conventionally impassable) fences in the way of clarification of the intuitive grounds of compulsory treatment.

It is not, however, an observation to go uncontested. After all, the idea that a belief which is true may none the less be a delusion is one which flies in the face not only of the definition of 'delusion' conventionally adopted in medicine, but also of that adopted in ordinary non-medical usage. In the *Shorter Oxford English Dictionary*, for example, the definition of 'delusion', "a fixed, false opinion with regard to objective things . . . " is closely similar in substance to the conventional medical definition. Indeed, the dictionary definition continues " . . . especially as a form of mental derangement". Moreover, to fly in the face of convention, medical and non-medical, in this way, may seem to be to abandon an important – Flew would say the only – defence against the misuse and abuse of compulsory treatment.

Yet the observation itself, that delusional beliefs, at least in so far as they are symptoms of mental illness, are not always false beliefs, is well attested clinically. The literature is full of examples of delusional beliefs (often of persecution) which were initially thought to be false but which subsequently turned out to be true. Some of these may of course have been misdiagnosed originally. But more than this, a belief may be identified clinically as a delusion even though *at the time* it is known or strongly suspected that it is not actually false. This is most often so in the paranoid psychoses, those psychotic disorders mentioned above, in which, often in the absence of any ancillary symptoms, the "best quality" delusions occur. The standard clinical example is the so-called Othello syndrome. In this condition, the patient, usually a man, suffers the (often highly elaborated) delusional belief that his wife or girlfriend is being unfaithful to him. So destructive is this belief, that even if it is not concordant with fact initially, it is often self-fulfilling. But in any event, as has been well recognized for many years (Vauhkonen, 1968), whatever else the diagnosis depends on, it is not that the delusional belief itself is false.

The Othello syndrome is not uncommon clinically. It is also important, with compulsory treatment in mind, because it is one of the few psychiatric conditions known to be definitely associated with an increased risk of homicide (Enoch *et al.*, 1967). The logical point, however, that delusions as symptoms of mental illness are not necessarily false beliefs, is made more arrestingly by those occasional paranoid patients whose delusional beliefs centre on the idea that they themselves are mad or mentally ill. One such patient was seen in a psychiatric clinic in

Oxford following a suicide attempt (Skegg, 1978). The patient
had tried to kill himself because, he said, he was "mentally ill",
and people who are mentally ill "get put away". In the course
of his assessment he was seen by three doctors, including a
consultant psychiatrist, each of whom was left in no doubt that
his belief that he was mentally ill was a delusion. Indeed, so
confident was the diagnosis that each of these doctors was
prepared to treat the patient against his wishes, should there
have been a continuing risk of suicide. In the event, the patient
accepted ordinary reassurance that people who are mentally ill
do not, for that reason alone, get "put away". Consequently,
although he refused further contact with the psychiatric ser-
vices, compulsory treatment was not thought to be warranted.
None the less, when last seen, the patient remained convinced
that he was mentally ill, and, by the test of competent clinical
practice, he was; for, by this test, he was deluded. But in this
case, at least, it could not have been the truth or falsehood of his
belief upon which this test, in the minds of the doctors
concerned, hinged. For had it been so, they would have been
faced with an impasse: to have considered it a false belief would
have allowed them to say that it was a delusion, but this would
have made it a true belief after all; and to have considered it a
true belief would have prevented them from saying that it was
a delusion, which would have made it a false belief after all.
More than an impasse then, a paradox – his belief if false was
true, if true was false.

It may now be said, but all this is rather small-print stuff.
That delusions, as symptoms of mental illness, are not always
false beliefs may be well recognized clinically. But whatever
the logical significance of this observation, whatever it has to
tell us about the concept of 'delusion', most delusions, if not
culturally atypical, even if not incorrigible, are at least false, and
more often than not patently so. However, there is a further
twist to the "delusions not being false beliefs" story which,
though less well recognized clinically, brings us (somewhat
paradoxically) right back to the mainstream, to the commonplace of everyday clinical practice. The twist is that delusions,
as symptoms of mental illness, far from always being false
beliefs, are sometimes not beliefs at all, or at any rate not

(falsifiable) beliefs as to matters of fact. They are sometimes not beliefs, in the dictionary phrase, "with regard to objective things", but *value judgements*.

This is most characteristically so in the affective psychoses, markedly negative delusional evaluations being associated with the low mood of depressive psychoses, markedly positive with the elevated mood of hypomania. In these conditions, indeed, delusions with mixed factual and evaluative content, are the norm – delusions of guilt, of worthlessness, of impoverishment and so on in depression; delusions of grandiose identity or ability in hypomania (see PSE generally). And besides these mixed forms there may sometimes be pure forms. Mr A.B.'s delusion that he had brain cancer was a (false) factual belief (though with strongly negative evaluative connotations). But another patient, Mr H., with otherwise similar symptoms, believed that his (actual) failure to give his children sufficient pocket money was a "deeply wicked" omission, a sign of his own "worthlessness" as a father and an indication that his family would be "better off" if he were dead. All, then, value judgements. Then again, Miss E.F., a novice nun suffering from hypomania, besides believing that she was Mary Magdalene reincarnated (a factual belief with strongly positive evaluative connotations), was convinced that certain small charities she had (actually) performed were of great moral worth: she also wrote mystical poetry which, though rambling and chaotic, she believed to be of unparalleled literary merit. Similar delusional evaluations may occur in other psychiatric conditions, in schizophrenia for example, and in organic psychoses, though less commonly, and generally with less marked and less unambiguous positive or negative colouring. They can also occur in the paranoid psychoses. Dysmorphophobia, for example, a "subjective feeling of ugliness or physical defect", may occasionally take the form of "a single, solitary delusion in an otherwise intact personality" (Thomas, 1984).

However, it is not really so paradoxical that this feature of the phenomenology of delusions, while commonplace clinically, should have remained largely unrecognized. The very oddity of the occasional true factual belief being a delusion ensures that it sticks out like a sore conceptual thumb. But for the conventional view, parblind as it is to evaluation, there is nothing similarly attention-grabbing about a value judgement being a delusion. Moreover, from a practical point of view, the two kinds of delusion, factual and evaluative, are so alike as to be identical twins. Of course, not having been differentiated, the possible practical differences between them have never actually been looked for. But this underlines their identity. For if the differences were there, and were in any way practically important, they would surely by now have been noted and explored. Whereas, as it is, in the present state of our know-ledge, the two kinds of delusions (for any given group of psychotic conditions) are (1) subject to the same treatments (the same drugs, the same psychological procedures – counselling, psychotherapy, behaviour therapy and social work interven-tion – being employed as appropriate in a given case), (2) carry identical prognostic implications (for suicide risk, recovery rate, likelihood of relapse and so on) and (3) provide equal intuitive grounds for compulsory treatment.

This practical identity, furthermore, has meant that even where evaluative delusions have been recognized for what they are, their logical significance has been missed, with evaluative delusions in effect being rolled up into factual delusions. For example, DSM-III is one of the very few places where evalua-tive delusions are mentioned as such. This is in line with the finding in the last chapter that evaluation is somewhat nearer the conceptual surface, it is somewhat more explicit, in DSM-III than in other conventional-view classifications. Yet even in DSM-III, delusions are defined primarily in cognitive terms *as* false beliefs. A delusion, the DSM-III authors say, is "a false personal belief"; it is based on "incorrect inference about external reality"; and it is held "in spite of incontrovertible and obvious proof or evidence to the contrary". Hence, coming to evaluative delusions, they continue "when a false belief involves an extreme value judgement", it is to be regarded as a delusion only if it conflicts with "an objective assessment of the situation" in such a way as to "defy credibility". Note, therefore, that word 'objective'. And if this is not sufficient evidence of evaluative delusions being rolled up into factual delusions, consider the two examples they give. The first (that one is "the worst sinner in this world") is indeed, or necessarily involves, a value judgement, but the second (that one is fat) is, or need involve nothing more than, a judgement of fact (DSM-III, p. 356).

Now, in this DSM-III conventional-view treatment of evaluative delusions, there are obvious echoes of the descriptivist ethical theory examined at length in chapter 3 in connection with the is–ought debate. This is only to be expected, of course, since the conventional view (as illustrated by Boorse) is essentially a descriptivist view (chapter 3). Moreover, the phenomenonology of delusions has important implications for the is–ought debate, implications to which we will return later. For now, though, notice at least that the rolling up of evaluative delusions into factual delusions in DSM-III is clearly analogous to the reduction of value to fact in ethical theory; and that, furthermore, in this respect the credibility defying evaluative delusions instanced by the DSM-III authors serve much the same purpose as the credibility defying normal evaluations instanced by descriptivist ethical theorists – namely, that of suggesting that at least for evaluations such as these, evaluative conclusions may indeed be drawn from factual premises alone. Here, however, by contrast, in developing a reverse view of the logic of medicine, a reverse, or *non*-descriptivist, ethical theory has been adopted: the argument being that even with credibility defying evaluations, any compulsion to draw evaluative conclusions from purely factual premises is not, as would be required for the descriptivist's reduction of value to fact, a logical compulsion, but, merely, psychological.

In a reverse view, therefore, as in non-descriptivist ethical theory generally, fact and value, 'is' and 'ought', remain sharply distinct. And this has the salutary consequence, noted at the end of chapter 3, that it brings us uncompromisingly "square on" to the ethical problems, practical and theoretical, of clinical practice. Which in this instance means that in a reverse view, value judgements as delusions, no less than true factual beliefs as delusions, stick out against the conventional definition like sore conceptual thumbs. The latter, true factual beliefs as delusions, showed that delusions (as symptoms of mental illness) cannot be (simply) the false factual beliefs of the conventional definition. But such delusions, occurring as they do only occasionally, could still, perhaps, in the conventional view, be discounted as rule proving exceptions. It could be argued, say, that the existence of true factual beliefs as delusions shows only that what is required for a conventional view account of 'delusion' is a sort of statistical version of the "implied cognitive defect" theory considered above. On such a theory, defective cognitive processes by definition normally lead to beliefs which are false, but this is not to say that such processes may not occasionally just happen by chance to lead to a belief which is true. So it is the probity of the processes by which a belief is derived, rather than its truth or falsehood as such, which is material to whether it is a delusion. And something of this sort seems indeed to be implied by those definitions of 'delusion', as in the *Oxford textbook of psychiatry*, in which they are defined not as false but as unfounded beliefs (Gelder, Gath and Mayou, 1983, p. 13).

The former, however, value judgements as delusions, are by contrast clinically commonplace. They are not as commonplace as false factual beliefs, perhaps, even (at least in pure form) in the affective psychoses. But they are certainly more commonplace than true factual beliefs. Not having been recognized as such, there are no actual studies of this. But as a measure of relative frequency, note that whereas delusional true factual beliefs are usually mentioned only in postgraduate books, delusional value judgements (without being named as such) are regularly included among the clinical examples of delusions given in undergraduate textbooks; for example, in Gelder, Gath and Mayou, 1983, p. 189, and in Leff and Isaacs, 1981, p. 61. No rule-proving exceptions these, then. And, taken together with the non-descriptivist separation of fact and value, the existence of delusional value judgements shows that delusions (as symptoms of mental illness) cannot be (simply) *factual* beliefs, true or false, founded or unfounded, at all. And with this conclusion, the conventional definition, so laboriously dismantled earlier in this section, when we were thinking of factual beliefs as delusions, now just falls apart. For, according to non-descriptivist ethical theory, it is only in respect of factual beliefs that the essential cognitive element in this definition, the element of appeal to evidence and to inferences therefrom, can be decisive even in principle. Hence, if as is suggested by non-descriptivist ethical theory, value judgements cannot – logically – be reduced to factual judgements, then, whatever the possible relevance of cognitive processes in respect of the definition of factual delusions, in respect of the definition of evaluative delusions they cannot – logically cannot – be decisive. While as to the incorrigibility of delusions and their cultural atypicality, the steadfast upholding of ethical convictions, even in the face of overwhelming consensus of opinion to the contrary, is traditionally a mark not of defective but of wholly sound moral reasoning.

But if being brought square on by non-descriptivism thus means, here, recognizing clearly the significance of evaluative delusions in showing the limitations of the conventional definition, it also, and correspondingly, means recognizing clearly the full extent of the difficulties involved in clarifying the standard intuitive grounds of compulsory treatment of the mentally ill. Indeed, at first sight, a non-descriptivist account of evaluative delusions may actually seem to undermine these grounds. Duff (1977) has made just this point in respect of the rather different case of psychopathy. Though it should be said straightaway that descriptivism, combined with the conventional definition, fails here completely – because the descriptivist reduction of evaluative delusions to factual delusions has the direct consequence that all those arguments (outlined above) showing the moral ineffectiveness of the conventional definition in respect of factual delusions, must apply equally to evaluative delusions. And this of course remains true whether a 'delusion' is defined as a false or merely as an unfounded belief.

When it comes to non-descriptivism, however, implicit in the non-descriptivist separation of value and fact is the suggestion, which as we saw in chapter 3 descriptivists have been quick to make, that *any* value judgement is in principle – that is to say logically – possible. *Any* value judgement, therefore, however (in DSM-III terms) "credibility defying". Hence, as far as logical constraints are concerned, non-descriptivism might seem to deny the very possibility of a value judgement being unsound, let alone of it being unsound in the specifically pathological way required to satisfy the specifically Hippocratic grounds of compulsory treatment. Furthermore, the psychological constraints, introduced by non-descriptivists in response to their descriptivist critics – in order to give substantive practical content to their moral theories (chapter 3) – serve in this instance only to compound the problem of the justification of compulsory treatment. For in speaking of psychological constraints, what the non-descriptivist has in mind is the marking out not of pathology, but of, say, immorality or criminality. What he has in mind is thus not medical or biological deviance, but social and political. Hare, for example, writes of "fanaticism" (1963b); and in a later publication, the (practical) answer to the fanatic amounts (merely) to consensus (Hare, 1981a). Non-descriptivism, therefore, in the case of evaluative delusions, may seem to drift perilously close to the view of the critics of compulsory treatment, the view that such treatment, so called, is really no more than social coercion wrapped up and disguised as medical intervention. And if this is so for evaluative delusions, the remarkable practical identity between these and factual delusions suggests, by extension, that it might be true for delusions generally; and if for delusions generally, then, delusions being paradigm psychotic symptoms, for psychotic mental illnesses generally; and if for psychotic mental illness generally, then, psychotic mental illnesses being paradigm mental illnesses, for mental illness as a whole.

Of course, any argument, non-descriptivist or otherwise, which tends to undermine the grounds of compulsory treatment, will also, and by the same token, tend to undermine the concept of 'delusion', hence that of 'psychotic mental illness', hence that of 'mental illness'. It is for this reason – it is because the justification of compulsory treatment of the mentally ill rests crucially on the concept of 'mental illness' – that critics of compulsory treatment are often critics of 'mental illness' as well (for example, both Szasz and Foucault). In this instance, however, in the case of non-descriptivism, the argument, although certainly capable of being read this way, can also be read in another way altogether. The critic of 'mental illness' can indeed take non-descriptivism, with its implication that any value judgement is logically possible, as showing that value judgements cannot be delusional. This was how the argument was read in the last paragraph. Read like this it tends to show that the concept of 'delusion', or at any rate that of 'evaluative delusion', is unsound. But the supporter of 'mental illness' can read the argument quite differently. He can take the non-descriptivist's demonstration that any value judgement is logically possible to show, not that the concept of 'evaluative delusion' is unsound, but that whatever it is that makes a value judgement delusional this has to be something different in principle from whatever it is that is involved in the logic of normal value judgements. If any value judgement is *logically* possible (as non-descriptivists claim), then *pathology* in value judgements (if it exists at all) has to involve something more, or over and above, the logic of normal evaluation.

To vindicate fully this supporter's form of non-descriptivist argument, the "whatevers" have to be filled in: whatever it is that is involved (conceptually) in pathological – that is, delusional – evaluation, and how this differs from whatever it is that is involved (conceptually) in normal evaluation. The supporter's form of argument thus requires some extension of established non-descriptivist ethical theory. We will be returning in a moment, and again in chapter 12, to how this might be achieved. But short of full vindication, notice first that what is required by the supporter of compulsory treatment, in extending non-descriptivist ethical theory, is no more (though also no less) than what is already actually implied by the (standard) ethical intuitions of everyday clinical practice. Indeed, the requirements of the supporter's form of non-descriptivist argument and the intuitions of everyday clinical practice are here exactly congruent.

Thus, the essence of the non-descriptivist supporter's account of evaluative delusions is that something more than merely normal disagreement in evaluation (however profound) is required for a value judgement to be construed as delusional = pathological. And the everyday clinical intuition with which this corresponds is that something more than merely normal disagreement in evaluation (however profound) is required to supply the specifically Hippocratic = pathological grounds of compulsory treatment. This was shown earlier in this chapter by the fact that in circumstances of mere disagreement in evaluation (between doctor and fully conscious adult patient of normal intelligence), the Hippocratic principle prescribes, not compulsory treatment, but, on the contrary, that the patient's wishes should prevail (in so far at least as it is their own interests which are at stake). This requirement, furthermore, as a requirement on evaluative delusions, is matched by a corresponding requirement on factual delusions, namely, that something more than merely normal disagreement on matters of fact (however profound) is required for a factual judgement to be considered delusional = pathological and hence as supplying specifically Hippocratic grounds for compulsory treatment. This second requirement (on factual delusions) is shown in a general way by false factual beliefs as delusions – Mr A.B., you will recall, whose mistaken belief that he had brain cancer was construed as a delusion, was treated compulsorily; but Mr C.D., who really did have brain cancer while mistakenly (but non-delusionally) believing that he did not, was not. But the requirement is shown also, and quite decisively, by *true* factual beliefs as delusions. Such delusions indeed are in this respect nicely symmetrical with value judgements as delusions. Value judgements as delusions show that something more than merely normal disagreement in evaluation is required for a value judgement to be delusional. True factual beliefs as delusions show that something more than merely normal disagreement on matters of fact is required for a factual judgement to be delusional. On purely clinical grounds, this symmetry should of course be expected, the two kinds of delusion, factual and evaluative, having identical clinical implications. And in non-descriptivist ethical theory it is there.

Short, therefore, of full vindication, short of actually filling in the "whatevers", non-descriptivism, read supportively, generates an account of 'delusion' which, in overall shape, exactly fits the intuitive grounds of compulsory treatment. It is thus a theory well suited to the issue between critic and supporter of such treatment. For it is a neutral theory, capable of coming out either way according to whether or not, in the event, the "whatevers" *can* be filled in. Furthermore, by taking at face value, rather than discounting, the full range of delusional phenomena – true factual beliefs and value judgements as delusions as well as false factual beliefs – non-descriptivism makes clear what descriptivism has tended to obscure, namely, just what a very odd conceptual species 'delusion', as a symptom of mental illness, really is. A clear recognition of the full oddity of the concept of 'delusion' is indeed a third thing that being brought "square on" by non-descriptivism means here. For in any non-descriptivist account of 'delusion', mere consistency with the basic data of everyday clinical experience requires that it emerge as a concept, (1) occurring in two distinct and logically non-interchangeable forms, as value judgement or as factual judgement, (2) which in either form is construed as such, *as* delusional, on grounds other than or over and above ("supervenient", for short) the grounds of validation/invalidation of normal value judgements and normal factual judgements respectively, and (3) which in both of its two forms, and notwithstanding the logical separation between them, carries identical clinical implications. The supporter of compulsory treatment, arguing non-descriptivistically, must show how it is that the concept of 'delusion' is like this clinically. Its opponents, no less demandingly, must show how it is that it only appears to be so.

So much is relatively uncontentious, a product of no more than the application of established non-descriptivist ethical theory to the established intuitions of everyday clinical practice. And if non-descriptivism thus shows that the concept of 'delusion' is odder than the conventional definition suggests, well, that is how things are. Delusion, as Mullen puts it in the *Essentials of postgraduate psychiatry*, "represents a profound and complex disorganisation of mental life stretching way beyond mere false ideas and mistaken beliefs" (Mullen, 1979, p. 40). It is the "profound and complex" nature of delusions which non-descriptivism – in bringing us square on – makes plain.

Yet we, here, can go further. We can go some way at least towards filling in the "whatevers". For with our extended reverse view, as developed in part III, we have in place already an extension of established non-descriptivist ethical theory of precisely the kind required either to fill in the "whatevers" or to show that they cannot be filled in. Our extended reverse view was developed by going beyond a consideration of the properties of 'illness' merely as a value term (as in chapters 4 and 5) to a consideration of its properties as a term expressing a particular kind of value, medical or pathological value as distinct from, e.g. moral and aesthetic. And it is essentially the same move which is required here. What has to be filled in is whatever it is that marks out a value judgement *as* pathological, and, correspondingly, whatever it is that marks out a factual judgement *as* pathological. Of course, our extended reverse view could still be wrong, notwithstanding the many useful insights into the logical structure of medicine it has already supplied. Indeed, so central are delusions, as paradigm symptoms of the paradigm form of mental illness, that if our reverse view were to fail to give an account of 'delusion', it would more likely be our reverse view rather than the concept of 'delusion' which is at fault. Though a positive result would, of course, secure both.

The next move forward thus has to be in the form of a hypothesis; three hypotheses in fact, one for each of the three conceptual fences in the way of clarification of the intuitive grounds of compulsory treatment of the mentally ill – the concept of 'delusion' (fence 3), the concept of 'psychosis' (fence 2) and the concept of 'mental illness' (fence 1). Testing these hypotheses will thus help to clarify the grounds of compulsory treatment. It will also provide a further test of our extended reverse-view analysis. Only an outline will be attempted here. This is a growth point for the argument, which like other growth points in earlier chapters requires much further detailed clinical and philosophical work for its development in full.

Fence-3 Hypothesis, re 'delusion' – *that delusions are (or are derived from) a species not of defective cognitive reasoning but of defective reasons for action.*

This hypothesis is consistent with, and to this extent it goes some way towards explaining, each of the three key features of delusions now displayed:

(1) *their dual presentation* Reasons for action, like delusions, may come either as statements of fact or as expressions of value. For example, if, while driving my car, I am asked why I turned a

particular way, I may reply either in factual terms – for example, "This is the way to so-and-so" – or in evaluative terms – for example, "I want (or need or ought) to go to so-and-so." This is true generally of reasons for action. Hence delusions too, if they are or are derived from defective reasons for action, may come, as clinically they do come, either as statements of fact or as expressions of value.

(2) *their supervenient definition* Neither all factual judgements nor all value judgements are reasons for action. Hence, something different from or over and above their status respectively as factual judgements or as value judgements is required to mark out either *as* a reason for action. Hence, if delusions are or are derived from defective reasons for action, it is in this "something different from or over and above" that their defectiveness would be located. Hence, whatever it is that marks out a factual judgement or a value judgement as a delusion – that is, as a defective reason for action – would be, as clinically it is, something different from or over and above the grounds of validation/invalidation of their respective normal counterparts.

(3) *their identical practical implications* It is from their status *as* delusions that the practical implications of both delusional factual judgements and delusional value judgements flow. Our hypothesis provides for this status to be located superveniently – that is, in something added on, over and above, their status respectively as factual judgements or value judgements. This does not guarantee that their practical implications will be the same, since the something added on could be different in the two cases, or it could be the same but with different effects. But our hypothesis at least makes it possible for it to be so: it provides in principle for *delusional* factual judgements and *delusional* value judgements to be, as clinically they are, two sides, and two logically quite distinct sides, of the same conceptual coin.

The need for further clinical and philosophical research to fill out this hypothesis has already been emphasized. However, that such research is likely to be productive can be seen by following a little where it might lead. Thus, an early priority would be to define in as much detail as possible the added on element of the definition of 'reason for action', that which turns value judgements and factual judgements respectively *into* reasons for action. Part of this, evidently, is a link (of some kind) with something done or proposed: in the example above, neither the factual nor the evaluative reason would have counted as a reason for my turning my car as I did if I had not so turned it. Another part, less evident, is a cross-link (of some kind) between the two sorts of reason, neither counting as a reason unless the other is implied: thus, "this is the way to so-and-so" would not have counted as a reason for my turning my car as I did if it could not have been assumed that "I want (or need or ought) to go to so-and-so"; and vice versa.

With the progress of further research, therefore, it would become clear that reasons for action, although indeed generally expressed either as factual judgements or as value judgements, are really cross-linked combinations of the two, combinations which are in turn linked to something done or proposed. Philosophically there would then be much work to be done in defining the nature of these links and cross-links, the constraints on them, their relationships to each other and so on. There would be much clinical work also. For with our hypothesis about delusions generally in mind, the philosophical work would naturally involve a critical re-examination of the phenomenology of delusions for signs of *defects* in these links and cross-links; breaches of the constraints, relationships which are not allowed and so on.

As to the likely success of all this, there is evidence in the literature already that the required logical elements, at least, are there. For example, it has regularly been pointed out that in the Othello syndrome the patient's behaviour – that is, what he does – and also his needs, are more important diagnostically in determining the status of his beliefs as delusions than is the truth or falsehood of his beliefs as such (for example, Shepherd, 1961, p. 690; Vaukhonen, 1968, p. 38, both of whom discuss delusions of infidelity in the Othello syndrome, which, it will be recalled, provide the standard clinical examples of true factual beliefs being delusions). Furthermore, if success is likely, then this is one area in which, besides philosophy serving medicine, medicine could well serve philosophy. For if delusions really are or are derived from defective reasons for action, then the clinical phenomenology of delusions represents an important resource of primary conceptual data upon which philosophy could draw in developing an account of reasons for action. Though this also raises the stakes. For if delusions really are or are derived from defective reasons for action, then philosophy, in developing an account of reasons for action, must confront the central enigma of delusional phenomenology – namely, that to the patient, his delusions, factual or evaluative, are not delusional at all. That which to others is most convincingly unreasonable is to the patient most convincingly reasonable. This is the central enigma.

Still, difficulties aside, the essential point is this, that in filling out our hypothesis with further philosophical and clinical work, the picture of 'delusion' which is likely to emerge is one which is *prima facie* fully compatible with our extended reverse view of 'illness': i.e., because an interpretation of 'delusion' in terms of defective reasons for action is *prima facie* compatible with an interpretation of 'illness' in terms of 'action failure', that is, failure of "ordinary" doing in the absence of obstruction and/or opposition. Both interpretations, of 'delusion' and of 'illness', imply an internal, rather than an imposed, failure of action. And the defect, therefore, which is implied by our hypothesis that delusions are or are derived from defective reasons for action, when it is combined with our extended reverse-view analysis of 'illness', turns out to be not just any defect, but a defect of that specifically morbid or pathological kind required to satisfy the specifically Hippocratic grounds of compulsory treatment. Thus, not only does our hypothesis account for each of the three key features of delusions, but, filled out with further clinical and philosophical work, it leads directly to a picture of 'delusion' entirely consistent with the standard ethical intuition.

Fence-2 Hypothesis, re 'psychosis' – that the concept of 'psychosis' is better understood not in terms of the conventional view of 'disease' = 'dysfunction' but in terms rather of our reverse view of 'illness' = 'action failure'.

The essential difference between the account of 'delusion' just outlined and that conventionally adopted, is that the former, instead of drawing mainly on the concept of 'disease', draws mainly on that of 'illness'. But delusions are the central psychotic symptom. Hence a similar 'illness'-based approach should help to provide clearer understanding of the particular kind of lack of insight by which psychotic symptoms generally are marked off from non-psychotic symptoms. The conceptual links between 'insanity' and 'action' have been remarked on in general terms in the literature: Edwards (1981) writes of mental health as "rational autonomy"; and Roth *et al.* (1977) include "rational reasons" among their proposed criteria of competence. In this section, on the other hand, a selection of particular psychotic symptoms will be examined with our more specific 'illness'-based hypothesis in mind.

The psychotic's lack of insight, as was found earlier, is at heart a lack of diagnostic insight. In the conventional view, however, diagnosis is primarily a matter of disease-diagnosis, of deciding the facts of a patient's condition, and, from these, the disease (if any) from which he or she is suffering (cf. chapter 9 generally). And this, too, is how the conventional view of psychotic lack of insight is best understood, primarily as a matter of lack of *disease*-diagnostic insight. In Aubrey Lewis's account, for example, there is the same emphasis on the facts. And it is this emphasis which allows him to assimilate what he calls the psychotic's "incorrect perception" of his condition to the incorrect perceptions sometimes not only of the non-psychotic mentally ill, but also of physically ill patients. As a lack of disease-diagnostic insight, then, psychotic lack of insight would indeed be, as Aubrey Lewis and those coming after him have claimed, no different from any other.

There is scope also in a reverse view for psychotic lack of insight to be thought of in this way. After all, the original sense of 'disease', that from which all others are derived, was analysed in chapter 4 as a particular kind of illness; and psychotic lack of insight is, as it were, a particularizing factor. It divides up mental illnesses into psychotic and non-psychotic. However, this division is *prima facie* a logically rather fundamental division, not so much because it divides the mentally ill into two classes – any binary factor, however trivial, does that – but because of the particular two into which it divides them; namely, those who take themselves to be mentally ill and those who do not. Hence, as a particularizing factor, psychotic lack of insight is one which we would expect to find operating well back along the logical chain of disease derivations defined in chapter 4, and, thus, close to the very origins of this chain in the concept of 'illness' itself. And if we scan the variety of symptoms traditionally identified as psychotic, this is essentially what we find. We find that not only delusions and hallucinations generally, but also certain symptoms of specific psychotic diseases, such as schizophrenia, have in common a particular kind of lack of insight which, though apparently so difficult to interpret on the conventional view, is on our reverse view readily interpretable in terms of the two-sided distinction by which the primary experience of illness was defined at the start of chapter 7.

The difference between the conventional and a reverse view of psychotic lack of insight can be summarized something like this. On the conventional view, psychotic lack of insight is, in Aubrey Lewis's use of the term, a misperception by the patient of his symptoms, as in the case of the acromegalic doctor who simply failed to "see" his deformities. On a reverse view, psychotic lack of insight is not so much a misperception as a misconstrual: the psychotic patient misconstrues something wrong with him either as something that is being done or is happening to him (the "illness versus done/happens to" side of the primary experience of illness) or as something that he himself is doing or has done (the "illness versus done by" side of this experience).

Take "thought insertion", for example, an important defining symptom of the major psychosis schizophrenia. Thought insertion is the experience of thoughts which are not one's own being inserted into one's mind from outside (PSE, no. 55): " . . . the thoughts of Eamonn Andrews come into my mind", said one patient. "There are no other thoughts there, only his . . . He treats my mind like a screen and flashes thoughts on to it like you flash a picture" (quoted by Mellor, 1970). Here, then, is no Aubrey-Lewis style misperception. The patient "sees" the symptom all too well. But perceiving it, she misconstrues it. Everyone else construes her experience as something wrong with her. She construes it as something that is being done to her. Not "as if" but actually so. In reverse-view terms, she lacks illness-diagnostic insight.

This comes out more clearly still in the differential diagnosis of thought insertion. Standardly, this is described in the textbooks as a two-stage process: stage 1 is the differential diagnosis of thought insertion from other similar phenomena; stage 2 is a differential diagnosis among conditions in which thought insertion proper can occur. Stage 2 is thus a straightforward matter of differential disease-diagnosis, the diseases in question being in this instance (in the present state of medical knowledge) mainly of the HDf3-type described in chapter 4 – that is, diseases defined by associations of symptoms: for example, thought insertion + clear consciousness = schizophrenia; thought insertion + clouded consciousness (that is, impaired cognitive functions, see chapter 8) = organic psychosis.

Stage 1, however, is better understood as a stage of differential illness-diagnosis. Thus, in the textbooks, which of course reflect the clinical situation, thought insertion is described as having to be differentiated on the one hand from the normal experience of one's own thoughts being influenced by others (see, for example, PSE, p. 160) and on the other from the abnormal but non-psychotic experience of obsessional thoughts (see, for example, Leff and Isaacs, 1978, p. 54). In illness-diagnostic terms, then, this differential diagnosis might be set out thus. The normal experience of one's own thoughts being influenced is like thought insertion to the extent that it is, in a sense, something that is "done or happens" to one. But the similarity is only superficial. For in the normal case, that which is being done or is happening to one is simply the *influencing* of one's thoughts; whereas in the case of thought insertion it is (bizarrely) the thinking itself. Similarly for obsessional thoughts, thoughts which, though unwelcome and resisted, come back repeatedly into the patient's mind (chapter 8). Here the superficial similarity to thought insertion is even greater, in that obsessional thoughts, especially if obscene or violent in nature, are often actually described by the patient as "not their own". However, closer questioning shows that the patient does not mean by this, as in the case of thought insertion, that the thoughts in his mind are those of some other agency. What he means is rather that the thoughts in his mind, although thoughts which he is thinking, are thoughts wholly uncharacteristic of him. And it is, on the contrary, this persistent inability to avoid thinking such thoughts (it is this failure of "ordinary" doing) which is at the heart of his construal of what is wrong, not as something that is being done or is happening *to* him, but as something wrong *with* him.

The differential illness-diagnosis of thought insertion is shown schematically in table 1. Presented this way, psychotic lack of insight shows up clearly as a mismatch across the "done-by/wrong-with/done-to" distinctions by which the primary experience of illness is defined; a mismatch between the way in which the experience of thought insertion is construed by the patient and the way in which it is construed by everyone else. In this table a further symptom, partial thought insertion (PSE, no. 55), is also shown. As is often the case, the partial form helps to bring out the logic of the full form. For partial thought insertion is the experience of thoughts being inserted into one's mind but from one's own subconscious. And this translates directly into illness-diagnostic terms as a sort of shift to the left in table 1: partial thought insertion, in these terms, is partial precisely because it is experienced by the patient in part as something done to him, in part as something he (the unconscious "he") himself is doing.

Similar accounts can be developed for a number of other schizophrenic symptoms. The central feature, for example, of each of the various "made" phenomena of schizophrenia, the so-called delusions of control, is said in the PSE (p. 167) to be that "the subject experiences his will as replaced by that of some other force or agency". One of Mellor's (1970) patients describes made actions: "When I reach my hand for the pen it is my hand and arm which move, and my fingers pick up the pen, but I don't control them ... I am just a puppet who is manipulated by cosmic strings." In the schizophrenic symptom of a made action, then, perhaps even more clearly than in the case of thought insertion, something one ordinarily does (moving), and something in the doing of which one may indeed be influenced by outside agencies, is experienced as something that is done *to* one. The "cosmic strings" described by Mellor's patient, stripped of metaphysical improbability, are, after all, existentially equivalent to someone (as in the example employed in chapter 7), simply taking hold of one's arm and

TABLE 1. *Differential illness-diagnosis of thought insertion*

PHENOMENON Thoughts in patient's mind	CONSTRUAL					
	By patient			By others		
	Done by ↔	Wrong with ↔	Done to	Done by ↔	Wrong with ↔	Done to
Normal	+			+		
Obsessional		+				+
Inserted (full)			+			+
Inserted (partial)			±			+

Legend: Psychotic lack of insight, in both full and partial forms of thought insertion, is interpreted in illness-diagnostic terms as a mismatch between the patient and others in the way in which the patient's experience is construed across the "done-by/done-to" distinction by which the primary experience of illness is defined.

moving it. And then again, as to the differential diagnosis of made actions, this too, like that of thought insertion, includes the (non-psychotic) obsessional symptom of compulsive actions.

There are of course difficulties with the symptoms just considered; and not all schizophrenic symptoms can be analysed in illness-diagnostic terms as straightforwardly even as these. Some of the difficulties are merely contingent. Thought withdrawal, for instance (PSE, no. 58), is the experience of one's thoughts being (literally) taken out of one's head, "sucked out . . . by a phrenological vacuum extractor . . . " (another of Mellor's patients). Something "done to", then, but something for which, in a differential illness-diagnostic table of the kind illustrated above, there is no obvious normal equivalent. However, this is not because phrenological vacuum extractors cannot in principle – that is, logically cannot – exist. It is only because, contingently, they do not exist. Other difficulties, though, really are logical in nature. But these, because of the kind and direction of the further research which is prompted by them, far from being prejudicial to the analysis of psychotic symptoms in illness-diagnostic terms, actually show its heuristic potential. Part of this potential, it is true, is more philosophical than medical. Thought withdrawal, for example, and, more so perhaps, thought insertion, raise in a peculiarly acute form the philosophical difficulties (mentioned in chapter 8) about thinking as something one "ordinarily" does. Indeed, the fact that made acts, more clearly even than inserted thoughts, are (as suggested in the last paragraph) analysable as "done-to" experiences, is itself a reflection of just these difficulties. We will return to this point briefly in chapter 12. But it is at any rate clear that these difficulties, as instances of more general philosophical difficulties, are nicely set up for examination by the analysis of schizophrenic symptoms in illness-diagnostic terms.

Another part, though, of the heuristic potential of such analyses is more directly medical. Thought insertion again provides a case in point. This is illustrated by table 2. Table 2, like table 1, is a differential illness-diagnostic table for thought insertion. Table 2, though, is an expanded version of table 1,

with another non-psychotic symptom added – namely, epileptic thoughts (normal thoughts and partial thought insertion
simply not being shown). Epileptic thoughts occur in the
course of certain kinds of epileptic attack. Phenomenologically
they sometimes closely resemble inserted thoughts. The two,
indeed, are often differentiated clinically mainly on the basis of
the presence of other less equivocal features of the conditions
(epilepsy and schizophrenia) in which they respectively occur.
However, an important difference between them is that epileptic thoughts, once their nature is explained to the patient at
least, are characteristically accepted (at least inter-ictally) as
arising from within the patient's own mind (Lishman, 1987; the
nearest equivalent to epileptic thoughts in the differential
diagnosis of made acts would be epileptic automatisms; Lishman, 1978, pp. 317–19).

Look now at the "wrong with" columns in table 2, "wrong
with" as construed by the patient, "wrong with" as construed
by others. These, too, have been expanded. They now represent the analysis of 'wrong with' (as illness) in reverse-view
terms as a failure of "ordinary" doing. The symbol " + o" thus
represents the reverse-view analysis of obsessional thoughts as a
particular kind of failure of "ordinary" doing, suggested in
chapter 8. This analysis, as was shown in chapter 8, has
considerable *prima-facie* validity, obsessional thoughts being
experienced by the patient themselves as being (in some sense in
which normal thoughts are not) out of his or her control. But
epileptic thoughts are also experienced by the patient as being
out of control. Hence, a reverse-view analysis of epileptic
thoughts in terms of failure of "ordinary" doing also has
considerable *prima-facie* validity. And if there are phenomeno-
logical differences between these two kinds of abnormal
thoughts – for example, epileptic thoughts being the more
stereotyped, obsessional thoughts the more resisted – well, this
is only to be expected if, as anticipated in chapter 7, they are, or
are products of, two different kinds of failures of "ordinary"
doing. Hence " + E" in table 2 is different from " + o". So
with the analysis of these symptoms as failures of "ordinary"
doing, a useful direction of research is established here. But the
real point of table 2 comes with the extension of this to inserted

thoughts. For inserted thoughts, unlike both obsessional and epileptic thoughts, are *not* experienced by the patient as his own thoughts out of control, but as someone else's thoughts altogether. So there is not quite the same *prima-facie* case for analysing them in terms of failure of "ordinary" doing. Yet the symmetry of table 2 is such that the direction of research established for (the non-psychotic) obsessional thoughts and epileptic thoughts carries through strongly to (the psychotic) inserted thoughts. Hence the significance of " + I".

There is thus established, by the illness-diagnostic analysis of schizophrenic symptoms, this direction of research – from a first interpretation of these symptoms in terms of the primary experience of illness, to their further analysis in reverse-view terms as, or as a product of, a failure of "ordinary" doing. However, what is of interest to us here, with compulsory treatment in mind, is not these symptoms *per se*, but what they have in common with other psychotic symptoms. It is what " + I" in this communal sense signifies, the particular kind of failure of "ordinary" doing (putatively) involved in psychotic lack of insight, that is the key to a better understanding of the grounds of compulsory treatment. So, before going into this directly, as we will in a moment under our fence-1 hypothesis, we will first see what can be learned about psychotic lack of insight by extending the direction of research now established for schizophrenic symptoms to the two general psychotic symptoms, hallucinations and delusions.

Hallucinations first: The standard textbook definition of hallucinations is along the lines of that in Harré and Lamb (1986); "perceptions occurring in the absence of an external stimulus to the sense organs", with a rider, variable in form, to the effect that they are experienced as real. This definition gives a standard differential diagnosis which, analysed in illness-diagnostic terms, nicely spans both sides of the primary experience of illness. This is shown in table 3, in the legend to which the various phenomena involved in the differential diagnosis are described. However, the feature of hallucinations of importance here is the one mentioned earlier in this chapter – namely, the dependence of their status as psychotic symptoms on delusions. This is implicit in the rider to the standard

TABLE 2. *Expansion of part of table 1 – Differential illness-diagnosis of thought insertion*

PHENOMENON Thoughts in patient's mind	CONSTRUAL					
	By patient			By others		
	Done by ↔	Wrong with ↔ = failure of 'ordinary' doing	Done to	Done by ↔	Wrong with ↔ = failure of 'ordinary' doing	Done to
Obsessional		+ o			+ o	
Epileptic		+ E			+ E	
Inserted (full)			+		+ I	

Legend: In this table another non-psychotic symptom, epileptic thoughts, has been added to the differential diagnosis of thought insertion, normal thoughts and partial thought insertion not being shown. Also, the "wrong with" columns now represent "wrong with = illness" analysed in reverse-view terms as failure of "ordinary" doing. The symbols "+ o", "+ E" and "+ I" thus represent reverse-view analyses respectively of obsessional, epileptic and inserted thoughts, as three different kinds of failure of "ordinary" doing.

definition, that hallucinations are experienced as real perceptions. Moreover, it comes out clearly when the sense in which they are "experienced as real" is filled out by their differential (illness-) diagnosis.

Thus, as can be seen from table 3, the sense in question is nothing to do with whether what is perceived "seems" real, for in this sense, illusions, too, "seem" real. Then again, although the required sense has something to do with whether the apparent physical properties of the perceived object are consistent with those of real objects, it does not have very much to do with this. A voice originating inside one's head, for example, though not a physical impossibility, is a contingent improbability compared with one originating in the outside world; hence, in the standard terminology, the former is only a (type I, see table 3) pseudo-hallucination. Yet many a conjuror's illusion is a good deal more improbable than this. One factor which clearly is important, on the other hand, is persistence, true hallucinations being very like normal hallucinations (see legend to table 3) except that they are persistent. The key is not in persistence as such, however – this is only the element of "intensity and duration" which is a component of any symptom (chapter 7). The key, rather, is in *what* persists, that is, not the perception alone, but the *belief* that what is perceived is really there. Without this belief, the persistence of a perception in the absence of a stimulus (if not "done to" = normal illusion, or "done by" = normal imagery) will be construed by the patient just as any other symptom is construed, as something wrong with him – that is, as a type II pseudo-hallucination. And that the required persisting belief is indeed, on the face of it, delusional in nature, is well shown by the way in which patients react to any contingently improbable feature of their (true) hallucinations. For the response of a psychotic patient to, say, being shown that there is no one in the room from which they heard voices coming, is not to acquiesce in the common (and most probable) explanation of his experience – namely, that there is something wrong with him – but rather to invoke ventriloquism or telepathy or simply to claim that the people who were speaking have somehow slipped away or hidden; or, if all these are impossible, that they are invisible. And this response, in clinical phenomenology (for example, in the PSE, p. 166), is actually called "delusional elaboration".

What is shown by hallucinations, then, is that psychotic lack of insight must be understood not merely as a misconstrual across the primary experience of illness, but as a delusional misconstrual. This is shown by hallucinations, and, once recognised, it is seen that it is also true of each of the schizophrenic symptoms considered above, thought insertion and the various "made" phenomena. Bizarre as the experiences involved in these symptoms are, it is not the experiences as such which are psychotic, but their delusional misconstrual as things being done/happening *to* the patient, in the face of the (surely) less improbable explanation that there is something wrong *with* the patient. Indeed, it is this latter explanation which, as was said, the epileptic "readily enough" accepts.

If this is true of all these symptoms, however, then why not for any others? After all, any symptom could in principle be (and most sometimes actually are) misconstrued across the primary experience of illness, so why not delusionally so? And this indeed, hallucinations, again, show to be so. For besides the (clinically paradigmatic) auditory and visual hallucinations instanced in the legend to table 3, hallucinations (broadening the range of symptoms which may be psychotic) can be olfactory, gustatory and even tactile. Furthermore, there is a class of psychotic symptoms which, though standardly called "somatic hallucinations", involve not perceptions but sensations – pains, vibrations, numbness, heat, cold, itching, sexual sensations, indeed any bodily sensation whatsoever. And the status of these symptoms as psychotic symptoms hinges not on how real they feel – a pain is a pain! – but on their delusional misconstrual as something which is being done/is happening to the patient. Leff and Isaacs (1978, p. 73) describe a variety of these symptoms, suggesting a screening test which involves asking not only "Do you have any unusual feelings in your body?" but also – making explicit the required element of delusional misconstrual – "What is it due to?" Their examples include "A feeling of thunder and lightning went through my arm", and "Crawly things run down to my feet"; or, with

TABLE 3. *Differential illness-diagnosis of hallucinations*

PHENOMENON	CONSTRUAL					
	By patient			By others		
Perception	Done by ↔	Wrong with ↔	Done to	Done by ↔	Wrong with ↔	Done to
Normal perception	+		+	+		+
Normal illusion		+	+		+	+
Physical disruption		+	+		+	+
Physical symptom		+			+	
Psychological distortion	±	+	±	±	+	
True hallucination	+		+	+	+	
Pseudohallucination I (in one's head)	+		+	+	+	
Pseudohallucination II (not real)	+	+		+	±	
Normal hallucination	±	±		±	±	
Normal imagery	+	+		+	+	

Legend: Normal perceptions are part "done-to", part "done-by" phenomena (see text here and in chapter 7), and the differential illness-diagnosis of true (that is, psychotic) hallucinations correspondingly spans both sides of the "done-by/done-to" distinction by which the primary experience of illness is defined. Thus, as shown in the table, this differential diagnosis includes, (1) *normal illusions*, that is, deceptions of the senses by some feature of the environment, e.g. the stick that looks bent as

Legend to Table 3 (*cont.*)

it is held partly immersed in water, the conjuror's illusion or the bush mistaken for a man at twilight; (2) *disruptions of perception by physical factor*, e.g. seeing stars as a result of a blow to the eye; (3) *physical symptoms*, e.g. double vision, tinnitus; (4) *distortions of perception by psychological factors*, e.g. the depressive who, anticipating criticism, perceives an innocent remark as critical; (5) *type-I pseudohallucinations*, i.e. perceptions in the absence of a stimulus which are experienced as real (see text) yet located as originating inside one's head rather than in outside space, e.g. a voice located as coming from just inside one's left mastoid process; (6) *type-II pseudo-hallucinations*, i.e. located as originating in outside space, yet not experienced as real, e.g. an alcoholic with repeated experiences of delirium tremens who sees snakes under his bed and is truly terrified, yet knows full well that they are not really there; (7) *normal hallucinations*, i.e., brief hallucinations; perceptions in the absence of a stimulus, experienced in outside space, and, at the time, as real, but then readily and more or less immediately recognized not to have been, e.g. the tired doctor who hears the telephone ring as he is about to fall asleep only to be reassured by the hospital telephonist that "he must have imagined it"; (8) *normal imagery*, i.e., images which, even if so vivid as to be experienced in outside space, yet differ from both normal and type-II pseudohallucinations in that, as the *Oxford textbook of psychiatry* puts it, they can "be changed substantially by an effort of will" (Gelder, Gath, and Mayou, 1983, p. 6). Note also, (i) that as in other areas of clinical phenomenology, intermediate and/or mixed forms of all these phenomena are common; (ii) that the table is not exhaustive; some might have included, e.g. hysterical hallucinations (unconscious simulation?) and visions (super-natural external stimuli?); and (iii) that there are many difficulties and differences of opinion even about the phenomena that are shown; e.g., some would include normal hallucinations with pseudohallucinations: these are differentiated here (following Hare, 1973) by the criterion of brevity, this being consistent with the fact that symptoms of illness generally are marked out from normal experiences by (*inter alia*) "intensity and duration" (see text and chapter 7).

more remote causes (the symptoms then actually being called "experiences of bodily influence"), "They work a machine which makes me feel an electric current passing through me." It is worth noting, by the way, that notwithstanding the standard definition of hallucination, there is no question of these symptoms being psychotic merely because of the lack of an appropriate external stimulus. These sensations are not, and hallucinations generally are not, in this sense simply "false" perceptions. Normal bodily sensations are of course not always associated with any clearly attributable external bodily cause. And as to somatic hallucinations, the sensations involved may, on the contrary, have apparent causes of an entirely conventional kind – like one of Mellor's patients who attributed the pain in his knee caused by a stellate fracture of the kneecap, to "the sun-rays (being) directed by US Army satellite in an intense beam which I can feel entering the centre of my knee and then radiating outwards causing the pain" (Mellor, 1970).

But if any symptom may be psychotic if delusionally misconstrued across the primary experience of illness in this way, what of delusions themselves? If a psychotic (i.e., "true") hallucination is, as it were, a delusional hallucination, is a psychotic delusion in the same sense a delusional delusion? Well, in a word, the answer, given the reverse-view analysis of delusions developed earlier in this chapter, is yes. For this way of putting it is really no more than a somewhat fanciful way of expressing the conclusion of that earlier analysis, namely, that delusions, as symptoms of psychotic mental illness, have to be defined superveniently, by something over and above both the factual beliefs (true or false) and the value judgements in terms of which they are expressed clinically. On this view, then, psychotic delusions include not only delusional delusions – that is, delusional false beliefs – but also delusional true beliefs and delusional value judgements.

Moreover, it can be seen now how this result, derived earlier by applying established ethical theory to the established intuitions of clinical practice, drops just as readily out of an illness-diagnostic analysis of (psychotic) delusional phenomena. In the first place, as regards their content, delusions fit nicely across the primary experience of illness. Most delusions are explicitly concerned either with things done/happening to the patient – for example, delusions of reference (PSE, no. 72), of persecution (no. 74) or of assistance (no. 75) – or with things done by him – for example, delusions of grandiose ability (PSE, no. 76) or of guilt (no. 88). And those that are not explicitly so concerned are still implicitly so. For delusions – at any rate the best-quality delusions of the paranoid psychoses – are never entirely neutral with regard to the patient. Even delusions about things apparently remote from the patient (for example, England's coast melting, PSE, no. 87) or delusions with no clear subject at all (called "delusional mood", PSE, no. 49) are experienced by the patient as "specially significant for him" (PSE, p. 158). Then, in the second place, delusions are, as the conventional definition implies, in *some* sense "false" beliefs. Hence they are in some sense *mis*construals across the primary experience of illness. However, delusional phenomenology itself, as set out earlier in this chapter, shows that the sense of 'false' involved here is quite different from that implied by the conventional definition. Conventionally, psychotic delusions are false beliefs in the sense that their content is counterfactual. But delusions, as symptoms of psychotic mental illness, also occur as true factual beliefs and as value judgements. *Prima facie*, then, the sense of 'false' in which delusions (as symptoms of psychotic mental illness) are false beliefs, has to arise from something "over and above" each of these. And something "over and above", furthermore, to which both factual beliefs (true or false) and value judgements *as* psychotic symptoms are related, rather as – in the illness-diagnostic analyses earlier in this section – thoughts, perceptions, sensations and so on, *as* psychotic symptoms, are related to "+ I".

Note, though, only "rather as", not "exactly as", since factual beliefs and value judgements *as* psychotic symptoms are a good deal more closely related conceptually to this something "over and above" than are other psychotic symptoms to their corresponding "+ I": *vide* the near tautologies one is drawn into in writing of delusions – "psychotic delusions"; this sense of 'false' that sense of 'false'; and the need a moment ago for the fanciful "delusional delusion" to express the illness-diagnostic parallel with "delusional hallucination". Yet this closer conceptual relationship leads straight back to our fence-3 hypothesis about the nature of delusions. For near tautologies are exactly what would be expected if this hypothesis, going as it did beyond established ethical theory, is correct.

Thus, it will be recalled that the fence-3 hypothesis was to the effect that the something "over and above" from which the status of delusions as psychotic symptoms is derived is no more than a (putative) structure of relationships and interrelationships between the very factual judgements and value judgements in terms of which they are expressed clinically. Hence, if this hypothesis is right, then although the status of other symptoms (thoughts, perceptions, sensations and so on) as psychotic symptoms would be derived from something logically quite distinct from delusions, that of delusions themselves would not be – hence the near tautologies. And this leads to a further point. For a main feature of our fence-3 hypothesis is the idea that it is by way of this (putative) structure of relationships and interrelationships between them that factual beliefs and value judgements become reasons for action. Hence, combining this idea about delusions with the direction of research established earlier in this section in respect of other psychotic symptoms, allows an extension of our fence-3 hypothesis from delusions to these other symptoms. For the direction of research established led to analysing " + I" as or in terms of a particular kind of failure of "ordinary" doing. And combining this with our fence-3 hypothesis thus suggests that the particular kind of failure of "ordinary" doing represented by " + I" is none other than that by which delusions are superveniently defined, namely, as suggested by our fence-3 hypothesis, a failure involving defects in the structure of our reasons for action. So, " + I" as used in this section actually equals "something over and above" as used in the last. But " + I", in what we called its communal sense, meant "psychotic lack of insight". So these considerations give a rather precise meaning to the observation from clinical phenomenology that delusions are the central psychotic symptom. And this of course carries with it the corollary (a corollary which also is consistent with our clinical intuitions) that the central enigma presented by psychotic delusions – that to the patient their

234

delusions are not in any sense false – is presented equally by any other psychotic symptom at all.

This, however, is one of those complications legitimately left for future research. It is the generalization itself which is important here; the generalization of the results of our earlier ethical analysis of psychotic delusions to psychotic symptoms, by way of an illness-diagnostic analysis of the intuitive clinical notion of psychotic lack of insight. The effectiveness of this generalization is well illustrated by hypochondriacal delusions, delusions of the kind suffered by Mr A.B. At first sight, hypochrondriacal delusions, perhaps above all others, might seem to endorse the conventional view of psychotic lack of insight, as interpreted in this chapter, that it consists in a lack of disease-diagnostic insight. On this view, the situation in Mr A.B.'s case was that Mr A.B. believed he had brain cancer, while everyone else believed that he did not have brain cancer but depression. However, as was shown above, this construal of the situation is inconsistent with the intuitive moral grounds of compulsory psychiatric treatment, since it fails to distinguish mental illness from physical illness in the intuitively required way. Also, and crucially, it founders logically on the paradox (which could be thought of as a sort of disease-diagnostic paradox) presented by the occasional hypochondriacal delusion of mental illness.

On an *illness*-diagnostic view, on the other hand, the situation in Mr A.B.'s case, drawing on the supervenient or "over-and-above" nature of psychotic delusions, was that Mr A.B. believed he had brain cancer while everyone else believed that Mr A.B.'s *belief* that he had brain cancer was a symptom of something (psychiatrically) wrong with him, that is, depression. This, as it were, second-order way of construing beliefs like Mr A.B.'s, besides being closer to intuition, is (strictly) implied by the existence of delusions of mental illness ("strictly", because it is necessary in order to avoid the paradox presented by a first-order construal of such beliefs). Moreover, this second-order construal makes it at least possible that the intuitive moral grounds of compulsory psychiatric treatment are sound. Though whether they are in fact sound, depends on the two further questions, (1) whether everyone else's belief in a case like Mr A.B.'s is well founded, that is, whether beliefs like Mr A.B.'s are properly understood as symptoms of mental illness; and (2), if so, whether this has the moral consequences intuitively claimed for it. Thus far, in analysing first delusions and then other psychotic symptoms, an affirmative answer has been given to the first of these questions. We now move on to the second.

Fence-1 Hypothesis, re 'mental illness' – that a reverse-view analysis of 'mental illness' in terms of 'action failure' is consistent with the intuitive ethical grounds of compulsory psychiatric treatment, where a conventional-view analysis, in terms of 'disturbance of function', is not.

To the extent that the specifically Hippocratic grounds of compulsory psychiatric treatment rest on the validity of the concept of 'mental illness', an affirmative answer to the first of the two further questions just noted implies an affirmative answer to the second. If Mr A.B.'s belief that he had brain cancer was validly construed as a symptom of depression, then, to this extent, his compulsory psychiatric treatment was justified. Further, the construal of Mr A.B.'s belief in this way within a reverse-view analysis of 'mental illness', has none of the counter-intuitive consequences of so construing it within the conventional view. Within a reverse-view analysis, there is no barrier to 'mental illness' having different moral consequences from 'physical illness', in contrast to the conventional view in which the validity of 'mental illness' depends on it being similar to 'physical illness'. Then again, a reverse-view analysis, as against the conventional view, gives a quite clear and definite sense to the intuitive clinical notion of 'psychotic lack of insight', a sense which, again consistently with clinical intuition, is rooted conceptually in that of 'delusion'. As against the conventional view, therefore, a reverse-view analysis has at least the right elements for it to be consistent with the standard ethical intuition restricting, as it does, compulsory treatment of fully conscious adult patients of normal intelligence, not just to mental illness, but (very largely) to psychotic mental illness, and to psychotic mental illness especially as constituted by delusions.

To the fence-1 question "why mental illness?", a reverse-view analysis can thus give what a conventional-view analysis cannot, an answer consistent with the basic data of clinical intuition. "Why mental illness?" ... "Because mental illness includes psychotic mental illness, especially delusional psychotic mental illness." However, it is worth adding that not only does a reverse-view analysis contain the same elements as clinical intuition, it contains these elements correlated with intuition in just the right way. The conventional view, it will be recalled, in so far as it acknowledges (by way of a logical double think) the concept of 'psychosis', requires that psychotic mental illness be at best no more, and at worst less, paradigmatic a species of mental illness than any other. And this, in itself a clinically counter-intuitive requirement, has the ethically counter-intuitive consequence that psychotic mental illnesses be at best no more, and at worst less, appropriately subject to compulsory treatment than other species of mental illness. All this, as was shown, is a direct result of the conventional view that 'disease', analysed in terms of 'dysfunction', is the (logical) root notion in medicine; thereby making (as in Glover's account) non-psychotic mental illnesses, such as obsessive-compulsive neuroses, closer parallels than psychotic mental illnesses to the (presumed) paradigmatic physical diseases. But in a reverse view, on the contrary, 'illness' is the root notion. Its analysis, furthermore, in terms of 'failure of "ordinary" doing', provides for a variety of equally valid species of illness, differentiated as different *kinds* of failures of "ordinary" doing (cf. chapters 7 and 8). And it is this analysis, applied now to psychotic illness, that gives results which are correctly correlated with intuition. For, consistent with the intuitive recognition of psychotic mental illnesses as paradigm mental illnesses, the particular kind of failure of "ordinary" doing implied by a reverse-view analysis of delusions (and hence of other psychotic symptoms) is a particularly fundamental failure. All other failures are, as it were, instrumental failures, failures in which the required action is defined but cannot (or cannot wholly) be performed – failures involving (in J. L. Austin's phrase cf., chapter 7) the "machinery of action" at the motor or sensory levels in the case of physical illnesses, and at

237

cognitive, emotional or appetitive levels in the case of mental illnesses. But the failure of "ordinary" doing at the heart of (a reverse-view analysis of) delusions is more radical than these. As a defect in the structure of our reasons for action, it is not an instrumental failure, not a difficulty in doing something, but a failure in the very definition of what is done.

One way to make this point clearer is to see how it might be developed out of the further research sketched under our fence-3 hypothesis above. That sketch went as far as the observation that an analysis of delusions as (or as a product of) defective reasons for action is at least *prima facie* compatible with an analysis of 'illness' in terms of 'action failure'. However, it requires only the results of the account given in chapter 7 of the kind of action involved in the analysis of 'illness' – namely, "ordinary" doing – to see that there is a good deal more to the relationship between these two analyses than mere compatibility.

Thus, it will be recalled that a key element of "ordinary" doing is intention. But intentions (as an element of "ordinary" doing) and reasons for action (as that from which delusions are derived) are intimately linked conceptually. Both, after all, are made up of fact and value (for intentions, see chapter 7; for reasons for action, see earlier in this chapter). Moreover, made up in this way, an intention *in* doing something can be logically equivalent to a reason *for* doing it. That is to say, intentions and reasons can be different expressions of the same (logical) thing, they can be logically equivalent in meaning. In the example cited above, in connection with the fence-3 hypothesis, my intention *in* turning my car as I did (that is, to get to so-and-so), was made up of the same logical elements, the same elements of meaning, as my reason *for* so turning it. From chapter 7, we know that for it to be my intention in turning my car that way to go to so-and-so, it must be the case (1) that I believe that that *is* the way to so-and-so (fact), and (2) that I want or need or ought to go to so-and-so (value) – just the same two elements, then, which, under our fence-3 hypothesis, made up my reason for turning my car as I did. But from chapter 7 we know also that one's intentions *in* ("ordinarily") doing something are a necessary part of the specification of what is done. Hence, to the extent that intentions and reasons are logically equivalent, if intentions are part of the specification of what is ("ordinarily") done, so also are reasons. Delusions, therefore, as, or as a product of, defective reasons for action, are, or are a product of, defects in the specification of what is ("ordinarily") done. And as such, not only are they, or are they a product of, a failure of "ordinary" doing – and, hence, in reverse-view terms, valid symptoms of illness – but they are also, or they are also a product of, a failure of "ordinary" doing more fundamental than any other. Analysed in reverse-view terms, delusions are thus consistent with intuition in being paradigmatic symptoms of mental illness.

This of course is to add nothing new about the defects actually involved, the breaches of the constraints, the disallowed relationships and so on, suggested by our fence-3 hypothesis. But it underlines how closely a reverse-view analysis correlates with intuition. Here, analysed as a failure in the very specification of what is ("ordinarily") done, is a sense in which the psychoses really do represent, in Mullen's phrase quoted earlier, a "profound and complex disorganization of mental life, stretching way beyond mere false beliefs and mistaken ideas". Here, similarly, is a sense in which the psychoses really are more "serious" than other mental illnesses (cf. the senses of "serious" implied by Flew and Glover above). Here is a sense in which the psychoses really are qualitatively different from non-psychotic illnesses, since the logical failure involved in a psychotic – that is, a delusionally-based – illness is different in kind from the instrumental failures involved in all other illnesses. Here, as a consequence of this, is a basis for the reliability with which psychoses are identified, since a severe and qualitatively different kind of illness is likely to be that much more reliably identifiable than others. And here, in the sum of all these characteristics, is a basis for the widespread recognition of the psychoses *as* species of illness, cross-culturally and historically, at least as far back as classical times. So that here, finally, in the correlation of all these intuitively recognized features of the psychoses with a reverse-view analysis, is a sense in which the psychoses really are paradigmatic mental illnesses, and mental illnesses, therefore, which, more than any non-psychotic illnesses, really do satisfy the specifically Hippocratic grounds required for compulsory psychiatric treatment.

In a reverse-view analysis, then, the right elements are there, and they are correlated with intuition in the right way. Yet satisfactory as this may be, it remains to be shown just why the particular kind of failure of "ordinary" doing (putatively) involved in psychotic lack of insight has the moral consequences it has. And this leads straight back to the central enigma presented by delusional (and hence also by other psychotic) phenomena. For while there is a clear general sense in which failures of "ordinary" doing justify the provision of help – help for those who cannot help themselves – and while this is important in the justification of all non-compulsory medical treatment, the fact is that the psychotic's own construction of what is wrong is, *ex hypothesi*, not in these terms at all. The psychotic, psychotically lacking insight, necessarily rejects the need if not for help, at least for help in the form of medical treatment of his symptoms. Indeed, the central enigma, defined earlier in epistemological terms, could be recast in moral terms as "that for which others are most convinced compulsory psychiatric treatment is justified, is that for which the patient is most convinced such treatment is not justified".

Yet recast in this form, there is an indication, at least, that a reverse-view analysis, while providing no easy solution to the central enigma of delusional phenomenonology, is none the less *capable* of providing a solution, and an interesting one at that. The indication comes from a different, but closely related, area of medical ethical difficulty, that surrounding the status of mental illness as an excuse in law – that is, as a factor, like accident, mistake and impaired consciousness, not merely mitigating an offence but absolving from responsibility altogether (see, for example, Hart, 1968). In this chapter we have been concerned primarily with compulsory psychiatric treatment because the issues raised by such treatment are issues familiar to doctors and other health-care professionals generally. But in forensic psychiatry and in law, the issues raised by the status of mental illness as an excuse are just as acute, and indeed in many ways parallel those raised by compulsory treatment.

Thus, mental illness as an excuse (1) has a special and unique status, different from all other excuses, including physical illness (Flew, 1973), (2) has been recognized as such cross-culturally and from earliest times (for example, it is mentioned by Aristotle in the *Nicomachean ethics*, Book 3; see Ackrill, 1973, Fingarette, 1972), and yet, (3) is subject to wide variation of opinion as to its proper scope and application (Walker, 1967). Moreover, as to the issues thus raised, the same three conceptual fences are found in the way of their clarification as are found in the way of clarification of the grounds of compulsory treatment. For if mental illness is an excuse, psychotic mental illness is especially so, and delusional psychotic mental illness even more especially so. In the Butler report on the treatment of the mentally ill in law (Butler, 1975), for example, of the six criteria proposed for the proper demarcation of mental illness as an excuse, no less than four involved delusions (the remaining two involving cognitive defect, relevant to conditions such as dementia and mental deficiency).

"Why mental illness?", then (fence 1); but also "why psychotic mental illness?" (fence 2) and "why delusional psychotic mental illness?" (fence 3). And at each of these fences, as with compulsory psychiatric treatment, the conventional view fails, and for similar reasons. It is recognized that the mentally ill are in some sense irrational, and that it is this irrationality which is at the heart of the standard moral intuition that they are not responsible for what they do. But the sense of irrationality involved has to be something more than mere cognitive defect – this is the central objection to the McNaughten rules (Hart, 1968). In the case of mental illness as an excuse, furthermore, this applies with particular force to delusions. Baroness Wootton, implying a purely cognitive account of delusions, has pointed out that, on this account, there seems no justification at all for excusing from responsibility the man who murders someone because he *delusionally* believes that he is being persecuted by that person, while hanging (as would have been the case when Baroness Wootton was writing) the man who holds the same belief but *non*-delusionally (Wootton, 1959.

241

Consistently, delusional moral beliefs, though possible grounds for a plea of diminished responsibility, do not satisfy the McNaughten test; Walker, 1985.) Sometimes this kind of case is considered one of "irresistible impulse". However, while the defence of automatism denies free will, there are no clinical grounds for supposing that the psychotic's capacity to resist is even partially impaired. In other mental conditions it may be – for example, in kleptomania, or pyromania, or psychopathy. But then the status of these conditions as excuses in law is considerably less secure than that of psychotic disorders. Nor is a more general conventional-view account, an account in terms of 'dysfunction', any more successful. For such an account correlates the wrong way with intuition. Boorse, in his version of the conventional view discussed in detail in chapter 3, acknowledges that his analysis gives the wrong result in this respect, the model of physical disease failing to explain the special status of mental illness as an excuse (Boorse, 1975, p. 66).

All, then, very much as for compulsory treatment. But in the case of mental illness as an excuse, it is more immediately clear why a reverse-view analysis gives the right result, allowing, where a conventional-view analysis fails to allow, mental illness the moral properties it (intuitively) has. For the factor common to each of the standard excuses – accident, mistake, impaired consciousness – is lack of intent. And it is just this that is implied by a reverse-view analysis of 'psychosis'. All non-psychotic illnesses, analysed in reverse-view terms, involve, as was said, instrumental failures of "ordinary" doing, difficulties in doing what one intends to do. And difficulties of this sort often mitigate and, if very severe, may even excuse. But in the case of psychotic illness, the failure of "ordinary" doing implied by a reverse-view analysis is a failure in the very specification of what is done. The psychotic, therefore, understood in reverse-view terms, lacks intent in that his intentions in what he does (or, equivalently, his reasons for what he does) are defective. In reverse-view terms, he is thus in the same position as others who lack intent in that he is not responsible for what he does, and, hence, excused.

Responsibility, however, is closely linked with rights, both intuitively and in ethical theory. Hence we come back finally to the implications of this conclusion in respect of mental illness as an excuse, for our understanding of the grounds of compulsory treatment. For, granted this link, if a reverse-view account of 'psychosis' explains so straightforwardly why the psychotic is not responsible for what he does, then this is indeed a clear indication that a reverse-view account should also be capable of explaining that most obscure of moral phenomena, the loss of rights necessary to the justification of compulsory psychiatric treatment.

11
Primary Health Care

Although in the present section diagnosis and treatment have been considered separately, it is clear that they are closely interlinked. The illness-diagnostic elements in the classification of psychiatric disorders outlined in chapter 9 are important practically because of their implications for treatment, mainly for what *ought* to be done rather than for what *can* be done, but important none the less. Conversely, the argument of chapter 10, although presented as an argument about what ought to be done, that is, as an argument in medical ethics, turned on the diagnostic difficulties inherent in the clinical concept of 'psychosis'. Indeed, chapter 10 could equally well have been presented (and actually did serve) as a detailed illustration of the points made in a more general way in chapter 9 – for the concept of 'psychosis' was explored in chapter 10 by drawing on the illness-diagnostic elements (of evaluation and of "action failure") outlined in chapter 9.

That diagnosis and treatment should turn out to be linked in this way is not surprising. It is well recognized that they are linked conceptually in their empirical aspects, sometimes, as with disease concepts such as 'B12 deficiency anaemia', explicitly so (cf. chapter 4). What has been added by the present analysis, therefore, is just that diagnosis and treatment are also linked conceptually in their evaluative aspects. True, the main carrier concept for this link is 'illness' rather than 'disease'. But then 'disease', according to the present view of the conceptual structure of medicine, is logically derivative on 'illness'. So the net effect of this view is to show that diagnosis and treatment are linked generally in medicine as two sides – indeed, as the meaning and implication sides – of the concept of 'illness'.

With this conclusion comes a shift, a sea-change, in the

overall drift of the argument of this book. Up to this point the argument has been analytic in method. It now turns out to be synthetic in effect. A common criticism of the analytic method in philosophy is that it proceeds by attempting to pull apart logical elements which in ordinary usage are normally not separate at all; fact and value, in particular, it is often pointed out, are in ordinary usage woven together in a continuous fabric. But it can now be seen that, taken to a sufficient limit, the end result of pulling apart the logical elements at least of ordinary medical usage – fact and value, 'disease' and 'illness', 'function' and 'action' – can be to bring them together again. And not just this, of course, but, to extend the fabric metaphor, it is to bring them together again with a far better understanding of their several contributions to the pattern on the cloth.

Mark you, better understanding, like better knowledge of fact, is no guarantee of better practice in medicine. Either sort of result, respectively of philosophical and of scientific research, can be put to good or bad use. Furthermore, the kind of understanding which is produced by the present approach, showing as it does the importance of the logical element of evaluation not only in treatment but also in diagnosis, places new and unfamiliar demands on the clinician. Whatever details are shown by future research, it is a clear implication of the view of the conceptual structure of medicine developed here that, contrary to the conventional view, there is always *some* sense in which (at whatever logical remove) a medical diagnosis involves a value judgement. Gone, then, is the (relative) comfort and security of the conventional restriction of the medical remit to matters of fact. Still, these new demands are already unavoidable. It just is a fact of clinical life that in addition to the empirical problems with which doctors are most familiar, non-empirical problems are becoming increasingly important medically. And it just is a fact of clinical life, therefore, that better understanding, in addition to better knowledge of fact, is an increasingly important condition of better practice.

Once the synthetic nature of the results of analytical philosophy is recognized, it is readily seen that philosophy of this kind has other contributions to make to medicine besides those with which we have been mainly concerned in this section. Better understanding of the natures of diagnosis and treatment, and of the relationship between them, brings with it the possibility of clearer, more consistent, and ethically more coherent principles of practice. This is an important, perhaps primary, contribution of analytical research to medicine. But a second, similarly derived, contribution is the possibility of better co-operation among the different specialist disciplines involved in health care. As Rachman and Philips (1975) have emphasized, the need for such co-operation in an age of increasing specialization has never been greater. Yet as things stand at present, the various health-care disciplines often seem openly antagonistic. The psychologist Eysenck, for example, has attacked, even-handedly, both psychoanalysis (1952) and psychiatry (1960). There is certainly a territorial motive at work here. But the scope for dispute is much increased by the lack of a common language. Each discipline has its own "model". Philosophical analysis, on the other hand, by showing the links between these disciplines, can supply a common conceptual frame of reference. Its effect, to return to the fabric metaphor, is to show how these various disciplines, with their different models, fit together within the overall pattern made by the medical concepts.

We have already seen two examples of this. At the end of chapter 7 the contributions to medicine of social and of biological science respectively were found to be reconcilable once the central place of the evaluative logical element in the conceptual structure of medicine had been accepted. And in chapter 10, law and medicine were shown to be fully compatible in their approaches to insanity once the derivation of 'illness' from "action failure" had been recognized. Other examples now spring to mind. Thus, this same derivation makes the relationship of psychoanalysis to the rest of medicine look less problematic, psychoanalysts being concerned with intentional and other "meaningful" aspects of a person's experience of agency. Complex philosophical issues are raised here (Farrell, 1981). But the point is that philosophical analysis, simply by highlighting the logical elements already present in the conceptual structure of medicine, shows this structure to be one within which, by whatever complicated route, psychoanalysis and, say, surgery *are* related.

Then there is mileage, too, without having to dip into the complexities of 'intentional action', in the two-way distinction (introduced at the start of chapter 7) by which the primary experience of illness is defined. Social workers, for instance, besides being concerned with "life difficulties" as causes and as consequences of illness, may also be concerned with helping people to see their problems not as things wrong with them – that is, as illnesses – but *as* life difficulties – that is, in the terminology of chapter 7, as things that are being done or are happening to them, and hence as things they can do something about. Behavioural psychologists, on the other hand, or those at least of a cognitive persuasion, fit across the other side of this distinction. They also restore agency. But they do this, characteristically, by teaching patients how to bring their symptoms – their anxieties, depressed moods, obsessional thoughts and so on – under their own control. "Cure", in behavioural psychology, thus involves patients ceasing to experience their symptoms as things wrong with them, and finding instead that they are things they can do something about. All these examples are rough and ready, of course, not fully worked out. But they show the extra conceptual elbow-room that there is in analyses of the kind developed here for different disciplines to work more closely together to the ultimate advantage of the patient.

These first two contributions of analysis – better understanding and better co-operation – are of practical importance mainly *within* psychological medicine. It is in psychological medicine in particular that non-empirical problems of diagnosis and treatment are significant clinically. It is in psychological medicine in particular that co-operation between disciplines with different theoretical orientations is crucial to patient care. But there is a third contribution of philosophical analysis, which is to give a more balanced view of the relationship *between* psychological medicine as a whole – with its several component disciplines – and physical medicine. I have written elsewhere of this balancing-up effect of philosophical analysis (1987). But it comes out clearly from the argument developed in this book. Thus, the argument has taken the general form of a stepwise transition from the conventional view of the conceptual structure of medicine, as portrayed in particular in chapter 1, to a new view, our reverse view. An important feature of this transition has been a change in the way in which the differences between 'mental illness' and 'physical illness' – in particular in the relative strengths of their evaluative connotations – are understood. In the conventional view these differences are taken as an indication that 'mental illness' is somehow a defective poor relation of 'physical illness' (chapter 1); whereas in our reverse view, on the contrary, they appear as direct and true reflections of the status of both concepts as equally valid subspecies of the general concept, 'illness'. This was clear even by the end of chapter 5. However, the steps in this argument, as will be seen in more detail in the next chapter, have been steps not so much of rejection as of addition. That is to say, our reverse view has been built up not so much by rejecting the conventional view as by adding to it a number of elements of the conceptual structure of medicine which, although always there, had been to a greater or lesser extent ignored: value has been added to fact, 'illness' to 'disease', and 'action failure' to 'failure of function'.

In the fabric metaphor, then, what has been shown by the argument of this book is that the pejorative assumptions about 'mental illness' (and hence about psychological medicine) inherent in the conventional view, arise from it being a view essentially of only one part of the pattern on the cloth – that part made up of the concepts most prominent in physical medicine, the disease/dysfunction concepts, with mainly factual connotations, outlined in chapter 4. The conventional view is thus an unbalanced view. And the effect of analysis, in showing up more of the pattern, has been to make possible a more balanced view, our reverse view, in which the psychological and the physical appear together as complementary parts of the conceptual structure of medicine as a whole.

Of course, even this balancing-up effect of analysis is a contribution more to psychological than to physical medicine. It works by enhancing the status of psychological medicine. Yet the main practical impact of all three contributions, in the short term at least, is likely to be not in psychological medicine as such, but in general practice and in other areas of what has come to be called "primary" health care.

The reason for this goes back to a difference in the logical natures of the respective clinical settings of psychological medicine and general practice. Thus, we saw in chapter 5, and again in chapter 9, that psychological medicine, at any rate in hospital practice, has developed essentially by following physical medicine along its path of specialization as a science. This has been an important and productive process, bringing with it, as in the case of classification (chapter 9), many successes. Yet these very successes mean that, even if the arguments of this book are correct, the illusion that medicine is nothing more than a science (the "science-based" illusion of chapter 2) may take almost as much shifting in psychological medicine as in physical. Not quite as much, perhaps, since the reality – the reality of the importance of non-empirical problems in everyday clinical practice – is that much more pressing in psychological medicine. Furthermore, it may well turn out that philosophical analysis has something useful to offer psychological medicine even in its development as a science. This point will be set out in more detail in the penultimate section of the next chapter. But what it amounts to is that philosophical analysis could help to establish a new paradigm for the development of psychological medical science, a paradigm less rigidly and unthinkingly modelled on that of physical medicine. And if so, this would amount to a fourth contribution of analysis. It would also be a fourth "synthetic" contribution, since, as will be argued in chapter 12, the most important way in which analysis points to this new paradigm is by showing the potential links between psychological science and physics. But for all this, the momentum with which psychological medicine is at present following physical medicine is such that it will probably have to get into a lot more trouble clinically before it is ready for any change of direction.

General practice, on the other hand, as an area of primary health care, is quite differently situated. General practitioners, interestingly, see roughly equal numbers of psychological and physical problems (Shepherd et al., 1966). They are thus in a position to derive at least half as much benefit as psychiatrists from the first and second contributions of analysis – better understanding and better co-operation within (mainly) psychological medicine – and, perhaps, twice as much from the third – better balance between psychological and physical medicine.

However, what sets the situation of general practitioners apart is that they see these problems (psychological and, indeed, physical) at a far earlier stage than their hospital counterparts. The hospital doctor, in physical medicine as in psychological, has the benefit of preselection by the general practitioner. This preselection is partly according to severity and duration of symptoms, factors which, it will be recalled from chapter 4, also select importantly for the (general) disease subcategory (Id) of the wider category (I) of illnesses. It is also according to speciality. Hence, since the specialities of hospital practice are scientific specialities, it is also according to the scientifically derived subcategories of disease, HDf1, HDf2 and so on, as described in chapter 4. So, all in all, the pre-selection by the general practitioner for hospital referral is strongly towards conditions a long way down the logical chain of derivation (set out in chapter 4) from 'illness' to increasingly specialized and scientifically based disease concepts. It is this pre-selection, of course, which allows the hospital doctor, especially in physical medicine but also to some extent in psychological medicine, to practice mainly within that part of the conceptual structure of the subject occupied by disease concepts of this "scientific" kind. But the general practitioner, although working to some extent in this area, has also to work higher up the logical chain, in the conceptually far trickier area of the concept of 'illness'. Mark you, even the general practitioner is not as far up this chain as the patient, for there are important selection factors operating long before a person goes to see his or her doctor – this is another area, the area of "illness-behaviour", in which analysis has something to offer, as was pointed out in chapter 7. But the general practitioner is a lot further up the chain than the hospital doctor. General practice is as it were wild-strain medicine. And primary health care, being in an area which is logically as well as practically "primary", is aptly so named.

Now, it is important to see that general practice is not thereby less scientific than hospital practice. Rather, it is more *medical*. That is to say, general practice is more medical in the sense that it deals with a wider and more representative sample of medical (and indeed other) problems, covering the non-empirical as well as the empirical. Moreover, it is important to see this both from an empirical and from a non-empirical point of view. From an empirical point of view it is important because it shows that there is no brief in this way of understanding the nature of general practice for any slipping of scientific standards. This goes back to a point made in chapter 3 in respect of medicine generally. Far from diluting medical science, a prime objective of analytical research in medicine is to clarify, and hence strengthen, the scientific remit. "Alternative" therapies in particular, such as acupuncture, must stand or fall by the same criteria as the products of, say, "high-tech" genetic engineering. For both, what matters is, do they work? This is (substantively) an empirical question. The fabric metaphor, again, is helpful here. To see more of the pattern is not to restrict or otherwise reduce the significance of its scientific parts. It is to get a better view of how these parts fit together with the rest.

From a non-empirical point of view, it is important to see general practice in this way – as *more* medical not *less* scientific – because it leads to a further potential contribution of philosophical analysis to medicine. This is a contribution more elusive of definition than the others, yet in the long run perhaps more significant clinically, and, indeed, philosophically. What it amounts to is a contribution to the repair of a certain kind of damage that has been done to the doctor–patient relationship by the development of medical science.

Broadly, it works like this. Medical scientific progress has been accompanied by a tendency for the patient-as-a-person to become displaced from the doctor–patient relationship, first by the patient-as-a-bodily-machine, then, and increasingly, by the patient-as-a-mental-machine. This is the damage. And it is extensive. Indeed, as I have argued elsewhere (1987), if there is a general cause lying behind the growth of non-empirical and especially ethical problems in medicine in recent years, it is just this machine "model". Such a model is appropriate enough up to a point for scientific research; it is appropriate, too, for the relationship between the doctor and the patient's body; it is appropriate, perhaps, even for the relationship between the doctor and the patient's mind. But it is wholly inappropriate for the relationship between the doctor and his or her actual patient.

Damage repair, then, involves finding a better model. But this, if it is to be approached rigorously, raises such conceptual questions as: What is the nature of a person? How are persons related to their bodies and to their minds? How are minds and bodies related to each other? How are different minds and different bodies, how are different persons, related? These are tricky questions, more tricky than any raised previously by the argument of this book. With these questions, indeed, we are brought firmly back to the deep metaphysics – the mind–body problem, the concept of 'person' and so on – from which we retreated in favour of a narrower logical analysis, in the strategy settled on in chapter 1. By the same token, though, these questions are indeed the very stuff of philosophy. Further, they are questions to which, once enough of the pattern is visible, the logic of medicine is clearly relevant: 'illness', it will be recalled, is unlike 'disease' in being connected logically with persons (chapter 4); so, too, unlike 'function', is 'action' (chapter 7). Then again, psychological medicine in particular, as we will see in more detail in the next chapter, is a source of much crucial linguistic data. Any philosophical theory of the person, for example, must take account of the clinical pheno- menon of psychotic lack of insight, that profound disturbance of the boundary between the self and the world interpreted here in terms of the two-way distinction by which the primary experience of 'illness' is defined (chapter 10). And if talk of psychological *and* physical medicine has a too unfashionably Cartesian ring to it, general practice, with its combination of psychological and physical problems, is the natural hunting ground in medicine for philosophical research directed towards reconciling mind and body. This in a sense would be the ultimate synthetic result of analysis, the synthesis towards which the other syntheses noted in this chapter are merely pointing. 'Action', after all, the concept at the heart of the present analysis of the logic of medicine, is bodily and/or mental (chapter 8). The synthesis, then, would be body and mind reconciled through the concept of 'action' in the concept of 'person'. And it is in general practice, in the wild-strain unselected clinical problems of primary health care, that this synthesis, as a potential contribution of analysis to damage repair, could first become actual.

It would be foolish, though, to overestimate the potential contribution of logical analysis to medicine, even in primary health care. There is no question, at one extreme, of all general practitioners, let alone all doctors, having to become philosophers! True, there are indications in the literature that general practitioners in particular are aware of the need for analytical research to fill out the conventional view. The need is not expressed like this. General practitioners are aware of this need from the sharp end, the end of practical experience. Hence, what is expressed is an awareness of the *practical* importance of the concept of 'illness' (for example, Helman, 1981; McWhinney, 1987); or, again, of the *practical* inadequacies of our current hospital-based classifications of disease (bodily as well as mental, for example, Jenkins *et al.*, 1985: though it seems that these classifications may also be inadequate, and for similar reasons, in certain areas even of hospital practice; see Mayou and Hawton, 1986).

But all the same, and even allowing for further growth in the importance of non-empirical problems in clinical practice, medicine, whether in primary care or in a hospital setting, must surely remain largely, that is in bulk or volume terms, an empirical pursuit. A large part of what goes on at present will thus continue to go on in the future, even if other (non-empirical) things start to go on as well. Then again, even where analytical research is properly appropriate in principle, the difficulties involved in carrying it through to a practically useful result remain considerable. As has several times been emphasized, all that can be done with work of the kind presented here, is to set the stage for more detailed clinical and philosophical research on specific problems in defined areas of medical practice. This stage setting, certainly, if it does nothing else, shows just *how* problematic these problems are. And this in itself can be helpful clinically. In everyday clinical work, it can come as something of a relief to find that at least some of the problems one faces clinically are, after all, not empirical but conceptual, and, hence, outside one's formal training as a doctor (given the medical syllabus as presently constituted). It can come as an even greater relief to find that some of these problems are, or are immediately derived from, deep metaphysical difficulties, such as the mind–body problem, which have evaded solution for well over two thousand years. All this helps to put in perspective one's relative failure to deal with these problems adequately in the contingencies of everyday clinical practice. But it also puts in perspective the likelihood of analytical research coming up with any quick results.

Yet it would be still more foolish, in the present clinical climate, to *under*estimate the potential contribution of philosophical analysis, to become too pessimistic about it all. The difficulties are real enough. But so, too, is the clinical need. Something has to fill this need, something has to address the growing importance of non-empirical problems in clinical practice, and it won't be science. It may not be philosophical analysis, either. But the potential contributions of analysis, even at the rather general level pursued in this chapter, are not insignificant: better understanding of what goes on in diagnosis and treatment, better co-operation between different health-care disciplines, a better balance between psychological and physical medicine, and better doctor–patient relationships. Merely to see what is required in order to realize these potential contributions, is itself an advance. To have come to see this from research into the evaluative element in the logical structure of medicine is an innovation. More detailed philosophical and clinical research is required to take things further. Psychological medicine, in which the non-empirical problems of clinical practice are most transparent, will provide much of the data for this research. But general practice, with its unselected and logically primary clinical material, psychological and physical, could well turn out to be the area of medicine in which the research itself is in the first instance most successfully carried through.

CONCLUSIONS

Part v

12

Overview and future developments

Scepticism has an important place in philosophy, provoking doubt, without which philosophical enquiry would not get under way, and providing a foil against which philosophical theories are most decisively tested. Scepticism about mental illness has served both these ends. Without the scepticism of Szasz and others there would have been no debate about mental illness. Without this debate the inadequacy of received ideas about the concepts not only of 'mental illness' but also of 'illness' and 'disease' generally would have remained largely unrecognized. Yet scepticism can have other less salutary consequences. Taken as too serious a threat, it can lead to dogmatism, a defensive hardening of conventional opinion – there is something of this in the debate about mental illness. Taken too seriously as a theory, on the other hand, scepticism can lead to a failure of intellectual morale, to a loss of confidence in the very possibility of progress.

Nothing in this book has been directed against scepticism about mental illness as such. Indeed, the overall form of the argument which has been adopted was suggested originally by the common ground between sceptics and supporters in the mental-illness debate. It was this common ground which showed the need for a far more thorough analysis than any yet carried out of the concepts of 'illness' and 'disease' as these are employed in physical medicine; and then for an extension of this analysis by generalization, rather than by direct comparison, to their use in psychological medicine.

Nevertheless, in the event, the results obtained have left little scope for scepticism, at least of any comprehensive Szasz-style kind. The view that the very concept of 'mental illness' is unsound – and hence that mental illness is a myth – relied on the idea that it was a concept prejudiced logically by the

difference between it and the concept of 'physical illness'.
Szasz, in particular, pointed, as many others sceptical about
mental illness have pointed, to its more value-laden connotations. Yet even in chapter I it could be seen that there were
no a-priori grounds for supposing 'mental illness', merely
because more value-laden, to be a defective – let alone a wholly
unsound – derivative of 'physical illness'. And by the end of
chapter 5 it had been shown, first, that 'mental illness' and
'physical *illness*' (as distinct from 'physical disease') were more
alike in this respect than had commonly been supposed, both in
particular being value terms; and, second, that understood *as*
value terms, the difference between them in the strength of
their evaluative connotations was no more than a direct
consequence of certain well-recognized properties of value
terms generally. 'Mental illness', indeed, in being the more
value-laden of the two, had been shown actually to reflect the
evaluative logical propeties of its constituents (anxiety, sadness
and so on), and to reflect these properties just as faithfully as
'physical illness', in being the less value-laden, reflected the
corresponding properties of its constituents (movement and
sensations). Hence, on this view, a view at this stage of the
argument already emerging as the "reverse" of the conventional view, 'mental illness', far from being logically
prejudiced, was actually endorsed by its more value-laden
connotations as compared with 'physical illness'.

On these grounds, then, mental illness was no myth. But if
the concept of 'mental illness' was thus not unsound, nor was
it, as its supporters in the mental-illness debate required it to be,
a concept just like the concept of 'physical illness'. As understood within a reverse-view analysis, 'mental illness' and
'physical illness' were equally valid species of 'illness'. But the
differences between them, reflecting as they did the properties
of their very constituents, were real enough. And this, somewhat ironically, although lending no support to the sceptical
conclusion, actually reinforced all those doubts and concerns
from which scepticism about 'mental illness' arose in the first
place. The tendency, among Kendell, Boorse and others writing in support of the concept of 'mental illness', had been to
seek to diminish the significance of the non-empirical problems

– ethical, medico-legal and political – with which mental illness, more than physical illness, is associated clinically. They had no option but to take this line given the conventional view – shared, of course, by their sceptical opponents – that the validity of the concept of 'mental illness' was dependent on its similarity to that of 'physical illness'. Boorse, it will be recalled, regarded these non-empirical problems, and with them the evaluative connotations of the concept of 'mental illness', as no more than a product of what he took to be the relatively "primitive", prescientific stage of development of psychological medicine. But our reverse view on the contrary showed problems of this kind to be integral. And this view thus firmly endorsed that part of the sceptical message which amounted to no more than an insistence that the difficulties inherent in the deployment of the concept of 'mental illness' be fully acknowledged. 'Mental illness', in *being* a difficult concept, was not thereby, as the sceptic generally went on to conclude, a defective concept. But difficult it was, certainly. And difficult, of course, not merely because of its evaluative connotations but also, as became plain with the extended development of our reverse view in part III, by virtue of its associations with that whole range of concepts – 'action', 'intention' and so on – involved in "ordinary" doing. Again, there was nothing here to suggest that 'mental illness', because of these associations, was a defective concept. As with its evaluative connotations, its associations with 'action', 'intention' and the like were a direct result of its very status as a valid species of 'illness'. And these very associations, indeed, once recognized, allowed in chapters 9 and 10 new insights respectively into the diagnostic and treatment difficulties raised by 'mental illness' in clinical practice. Not a defective concept, then, the concept of 'mental illness', just difficult. But difficult in ways and to an extent that set it apart, as a concept quite different from the concept of 'physical illness'.

Neither side, therefore, neither sceptic nor supporter in the debate about 'mental illness', has been endorsed by the reverse view of the logical structure of medicine developed in this book. Not, though, that in this instance, this gives grounds for any loss of intellectual morale. For, if both sides in the mental-illness debate are wrong, it is nonetheless, as has been said, through the debate itself that progress has been made possible – the assumptions common to sceptic and supporter, their shared conventional view, having been made plain by the debate between them, and the failure of *both* their positions thus leading directly to the development of a view which is indeed no less than the reverse of their conventional view.

Thesis plus antithesis has thus led to a new synthesis. And as to this new synthesis, so inclusive has it proved to be, that its basic themes at least can surely now no longer be resisted. The basic themes in any conventional-view theory are, first, that the conceptual structure of medicine is essentially factual in nature, and, second, that this is so because a biological-scientific concept of 'disease', defined in terms of a (supposedly) value-free concept of 'dysfunction', is logically central in medicine. The theories of Szasz, Kendell and Boorse, it will be recalled, were all built on these two themes. But the corresponding basic themes of the theory developed in this book are (in the sense of the term as it has been used here) the reverse of these. They are, first, that the conceptual structure of medicine is essentially evaluative (rather than factual) in nature, and, second, that the particular kind of value which is expressed by medical terms is derived via 'illness' (rather than 'disease') from 'failure of action' (rather than 'failure of function'). These reverse-view themes are, perhaps, *prima facie* less plausible than their conventional-view counterparts. They are after all not self-evident. They have had to be dug for. Furthermore, in their detailed working out in this book, there is no doubt much with which it is possible to find fault. Certainly, this working out – though this is no fault – is in places incomplete, at the many "growth points" for the argument noted in passing. But then it is results which count. And the plain fact is that the model of the conceptual structure of medicine built up here on these reverse-view themes, imperfect and incomplete as it may be, correlates with and illuminates ordinary medical usage at many more points than any model that has yet been built on the superficially more plausible conventional-view themes. (A summary comparison of conventional- and reverse-view analyses of the medical concepts is given in tabular form in the appendix.)

With hindsight it can be seen that there are good philosophical reasons, to do with the broadly Wittgensteinian approach adopted in chapter 1, for the success of our reverse view. The conventional view, as the basis of the positions of both sceptic and supporter in the debate about mental illness, is really a view of medicine as a science. It is, as it was called in chapter 2, a medical-scientific view. This science-based view is natural enough, given the importance of science in medicine. However, developed in any detail, it runs into all the conceptual difficulties noted in chapter 2 and succeeding chapters. The conventional response to these difficulties has been to seek to improve and refine further the science-based view of medicine. This is Boorse's response, for example. Nor is there any a-priori reason why this kind of response should fail. But so far it has failed. The alternative, Wittgenstein-led response is to suspect that the difficulties encountered in developing a science-based view of medicine arise from, and are therefore themselves evidence of, that view being a too restricted view of medicine. Wittgenstein, it will be recalled, suggested that philosophical problems generally were of this nature. He argued that they were difficulties created by a kind of philosophical tunnel vision, by philosophers taking too narrow or too one-sided a view of the concepts with which they were concerned. And this is what the conventional science-based view of medicine can now be seen to have been. Whereas our reverse view – which is by contrast an ethics-based view of medicine – is in its more comprehensive correlation with ordinary medical usage a view which encompasses, but is not restricted to, the nature of medicine as a science.

The very name "reverse" has thus turned out to have been something of a misnomer. Appropriate enough as the argument was developing – in that it emphasized the way in which each key feature of the new view as it emerged proved to be the reverse of its conventional-view counterpart – but failing to capture the full scope of the end product as, in this Wittgensteinian sense, a more whole or complete view of medicine. And if it has taken hindsight to see the new view in this way, this is because of the somewhat circuitous route by which we have come to it. It would certainly have been possible to have gone more directly to an ethics-based end product. A simple outlining of the deficiencies in existing science-based views of medicine could have suggested, on the Wittgensteinian grounds just noted, the need for a more whole view. And what more obvious than to look for such a view in the ethical, as distinct from the scientific, parts of the subject.

This direct route, however, would have left too much scope for the conventional response to the recognition of deficiencies in the science-based view. It would have left too much room for the belief that what was needed was not an ethics-based view, nor any other kind of non-scientific view, but rather an improved science-based view. Hence the route taken here has been to seek first to undermine the grounds of science-based views in general and only then to go on to develop an ethics-based view. Most of this undermining was done in chapter 3. In that chapter an imaginary descriptivist versus non-descriptivist debate about Boorse's theory was used to show that even the biological-scientific concept of 'dysfunction' could not be defined (as required by all science-based theories) value-free; or, to be more exact, that if 'dysfunction' *were* so defined, it could not then do the job which it actually does do, and which Boorse, despite himself, actually continued to make it do, in the logical structure of medicine. This then left the way clear for analyses of 'disease' and 'illness', respectively in chapters 4 and 5, *as* value terms. However, successful as these analyses turned out to be, it was only when we went on to consider the particular kind of value expressed by these terms that really useful analyses of 'mental illness' became possible. Here again the first step was a consideration of 'dysfunction'. An apparent loophole which had been left in the argument of chapter 3 was picked up in chapter 6 and shown to lead directly to the result that the evaluative element in the meaning of 'dysfunction' was derived from 'intention'. This result then led in chapter 7 to a substantive analysis of 'illness' in terms of its logical origins in 'failure of action', and so to the full spread of results for 'mental illness' in chapters 8–10, and for medicine generally in chapter 11.

The end product, then, the ethics-based view of the logical structure of medicine developed here, is this. In medicine, just as illness – the patient's direct experience of something wrong –

normally precedes a clinical diagnosis of *what* is wrong in terms of particular diseases, so, in the logic of medicine it is 'illness' which comes first. Science is important in medicine, and empirically derived disease concepts are correspondingly prominent in ordinary medical usage. But the order of logical derivation is not 'disease' first then 'illness', but 'illness' first then 'disease'. 'Illness' itself is then in turn derived from 'action failure'. Specifically, its logical origins are to be found in the experience of failure of "ordinary" doing in the perceived absence of obstruction and/or opposition – "action failure" for short. It is in terms of these origins that the logical properties of 'illness', and hence indirectly also of 'disease' and other related concepts, are to be understood.

Thus, from the "action" in 'action failure' come many of the general properties of 'illness': its special link with persons, its vagueness, its subjectivity and also, because of the intentionality latent in "ordinary" doing, its properties as a value term. It is one of these evaluative properties which is crucial to the derivation of 'disease', namely, the negative correlation which exists between the strength of the evaluative connotations of a value term and the extent to which the criteria for the application of that term are settled or agreed upon. This negative correlation ensures that 'disease' in its logically primitive sense (defined in chapter 4) as "a condition widely regarded as an illness" has mainly factual connotations. And from this primitive sense the whole structure of relatively value-free disease concepts so prominent in ordinary medical usage can be derived – as historically they were derived – by the play of straightforwardly empirical factors operating under the selective pressures of clinical utility. From the "failure" in 'action failure', on the other hand, come all the more specific properties of 'illness' as a term expressing a particular kind of value, negative medical value as distinct from moral or aesthetic value. It is this "action *failure*", for example, that makes illness an excuse ('ought' implying 'can'). It is this, too, that links 'illness' with 'dysfunction' (this link being the obverse of that between 'action' and 'function'). And it is this, above all, that, given the diversity of possible kinds of action failure, generates the diversity of illness concepts by which the (overlapping)

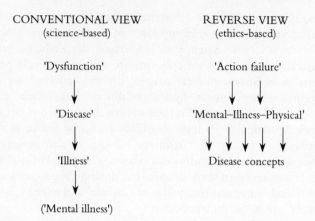

FIGURE I *Comparison of conventional and reverse views of the conceptual structure of medicine*
In the conventional view, failure of function, or 'dysfunction', is the logical root notion. 'Illness' is derived from 'disease' which in turn is derived from 'dysfunction'. Also, 'mental illness' is more remote logically than 'physical illness' from what is taken to be the paradigmatic 'disease = dysfunction'. In the view developed here, on the other hand, the relationship between 'illness' and 'disease' is reversed. 'Disease' is derived from 'illness', not 'illness' from 'disease'. This reverse view is consistent with the existence of a range of mental and physical concepts of illness and disease equidistant logically from their common conceptual origins in the experience of "action failure".

concepts of 'mental illness' and 'physical illness' are comprised in ordinary medical usage.

But what of clinical utility? After all, the extent to which this new ethics-based view correlates with and explains ordinary medical usage, constitutes good but only first outcome criterion support for it. And clinical utility, as a second outcome criterion, is, as will be recalled from chapter I, its more acid test. Yet clinical utility has been relatively neglected here. To some extent this has been inevitable. Theory and practice are like chicken and egg. Over a period of time each begets the other. But in medicine now – and this is the starting point for this book – there are many more clinically problematic eggs than satisfactory theoretical hens. Hence the priority has been theory rather than practice. However, as we saw in chapter I, it is precisely because theory in this area has been begotten of practice – the whole debate about 'mental illness' and hence about the concepts of 'illness' and 'disease' generally having been prompted by clinical difficulties – it is for precisely this reason that clinical utility is inescapably an outcome criterion for work of this kind. It is important to be clear on this point. What is at issue is not a cost–benefit analysis of the kind appropriate to, say, cancer research. Epigrammatically, there is more to life than limb. What is at issue, rather, is theory itself. Clinical utility, important as it is in its own right, is of interest here for the indication it gives of the probity of theory.

Not, though, that clinical utility has been wholly ignored here. On the contrary, chapter 5, and to a greater extent each of the chapters in part IV, were applied chapters. And in all these chapters the new ethics-based view was found to illuminate important areas of clinical difficulty. Again, as with its ability to explain ordinary medical usage, there was a certain Wittgensteinian logic to the successes of the new view in respect of these clinical difficulties. For the difficulties in question, being difficulties of the kind which gave rise to the mental-illness debate, are not empirical difficulties but *non*-empirical. As discussed in chapter I, the difficulties in medical practice with which work of this kind is concerned are primarily conceptual difficulties, both in their own right and as underlying ethical, medico-legal and political clinical problems. Hence, not only is this new ethics-based view broader in a Wittgensteinian sense than any science-based view, it is also broader in a respect directly apposite to the particular kind of clinical difficulties from which it sprang, and towards which, in its theoretical aspects, it is primarily directed. It is true that much of the contents of chapter 5 and part IV went towards illuminating and extending the theory. But this is how it should be. For in the course of this a framework was established, and a number of specific "growth points" were identified, for new clinical and philosophical research directed towards more substantive practical results. Much more than this a general theory, of its nature, cannot supply. Substantive results require substantive research.

However, without attempting to anticipate in detail the results of future research, it is possible to speculate in outline on the kinds of direction such research might take, and hence on some of the developments in medicine to which work of the sort presented in this book might lead. It is with these speculations, first in science, then in philosophy, that the remainder of this chapter will be concerned.

Medicine and science

Notwithstanding the development of the present ethics-based view of the logical structure of medicine as the "reverse" of conventional science-based views, a recurring theme in this book has been the sympathy which exists between science and ethics in medicine. At the conclusion of the debate in chapter 3, the non-descriptivist philosopher argued that to acknowledge the existence of an irreducibly evaluative element in the meanings of terms such as 'illness' and 'disease', far from rendering impossible Boorse's objective of a value-free science of health, actually clarifies the remit of such a science as essentially descriptive, like the remit of any other science. This conclusion came out clearly in chapter 6, in which the biological-scientific concept of 'dysfunction', so central to conventional science-based views, was considered in more detail. In principle, the scientific account of biological bodies could be given in terms no different from that of non-biological bodies – livers and lungs like rivers and suns. In fact, however, the scientific account of biological bodies is in functional, hence teleological, hence value-laden terms. According to the argument of chapter 6, to add to the language of cause and effect the language of means and ends, is to add to a description of what is done an account of why it is done, and, hence, the value-laden notion of intention. But the point is that if a functional account of biological bodies thus entails evaluation as well as description, the descriptive part of such an account, its properly scientific part, is no less "scientific" for that.

In the present case the contrast implied by calling our developing ethics-based view a "reverse" view was necessary – or at any rate intended – as a jolt to dispel what is in effect an illusion, the conventional science-based illusion that medicine, if it is not *just* a science, is at any rate at *heart* a science. Bred on the success of science in medicine, this is an illusion to which, as Farrell has remarked (1979), doctors actively cling. Yet it would be ironic if in the future development of the relationship between medicine and science, this science-based illusion were merely to be replaced by another – by an ethics-based illusion, the illusion that medicine, because it is not *just* a science, is thus any *less* of a science. What is required, then, is not another illusion, another one-sided view of medicine, but a more balanced view, a view in which both evaluative and descriptive elements in the logical structure of the subject are fully acknowledged. And to the extent that the present theory contributes to the development of such a view, its effect should be not to diminish but to clarify the place of science in medicine, and thus not to inhibit but to promote medical scientific progress.

This much, then, has been said already. But to these somewhat negative considerations can now be added others more positive. In respect of physical medicine, it is perhaps sufficient to say of an ethics-based view that its dissemination will not interfere with the development of medical science; that, on the contrary, it will "clear the path" as it were. But in respect of psychological medicine an ethics-based view may also have a more active role to play in promoting scientific advance. There are two reasons for believing this to be so, one not too speculative, the other more speculative but also more intriguing. Both arise generally from the greater conceptual difficulty of psychological medicine compared with physical medicine and the corresponding greater conceptual difficulty of mental science compared with bodily science.

Thus, the first reason, the not too speculative reason, has to do with 'disease'. It comes from the way in which, on an ethics-based view of medicine, disease concepts are derived from 'illness'. It is in the development of disease concepts in physical medicine that medical science has been most spectacularly successful. One effect of this success has been the widespread assumption, noted in chapter 5, that psychological disease concepts should be modelled directly on physical. Yet, as was pointed out, once the derivative nature of 'disease' is recognized, it becomes clear that this assumption could well be overly restrictive. And in chapter 9, in which problems of psychiatric diagnosis were reviewed, this was indeed found to be so. The main point made in chapter 9, however, was the rather general one that non-empirical (as well as empirical) factors are important in the classification of psychiatric disorders in ways and to an extent that they are not in the classification of physical disorders – essentially because the value-laden concept of 'illness' (as well as the more factual 'disease') is important and problematic in the everyday practice of psychological medicine in ways and to an extent that it is not in the practice of physical medicine.

The point to be made here, on the other hand, though based on similar considerations, is for science itself. It is that once the derivative nature of 'disease' is recognized, it becomes natural to think of psychological disease concepts, even in their purely *empirical* aspects, as developing, not along the same lines as physical, but along distinct branches of (albeit) the same family tree. The point is made graphically by the figure given earlier in this chapter. This is a model for scientific innovation. In just what such innovation might consist, it is the job of future scientific work to discover. But at the very least, an ethics-based view, by establishing the derivation of 'disease' from 'illness', frees up the imagination to new possibilities. In default, there will remain good practical reasons for following Wing's advice (1978) and concentrating on those psychological disorders most closely analogous to physical disorders; for it is here that the established techniques and ideas of physical medicine can be transposed to psychological medicine with the best chance of success – Wing had in mind the psychoses especially. But an ethics-based view, as a view fully open to opportunities for scientific innovation, supplies an essential ground of progress in psychological medicine, and, hence, and importantly, in the psychological sciences relevant to it.

The second, more speculative reason for believing that an ethics-based view has a positive role to play in promoting scientific advance has to do with the concept of 'illness'. Unlike the first reason, which has to do merely with mental set, this reason has to do with the actual direction of future scientific advance. Hence its more speculative nature. It arises from the fact that in the ethics-based view developed here, and indeed in ordinary usage, the concept of 'disease', as the main carrier of the empirical content of medicine, is not sharply distinct from the concept of 'illness' – 'illness' filtering through into and providing the logical framework within which disease concepts have developed. It has been convenient in places to write of 'illness' and 'disease' as though they were quite distinct. In chapter 4, in particular, the features of ordinary medical usage were built up by addition, by summation across a variety of hypothetical distinct concepts – 'illness', defined by the category "I", and not just 'disease', but a whole series of disease concepts, HDf1, HDf2 and so on, based on the subcategory "Id". Yet in ordinary medical usage, as was emphasized in chapter 4, 'disease', in its various forms, and 'illness' are not sharply distinct in this way. This observation may have little consequence for science in physical medicine, in which 'illness' is not very prominent. But in psychological medicine its effect is to suggest that the concepts from which 'illness' itself is derived could be important, via the logical connection between 'illness' and 'disease', *scientifically*. Not merely, then, the concepts of 'dysfunction' and 'function', as in the conventional science-based view, but 'failure of action' and 'action'. What is implied, therefore, by the observation that the concepts of 'disease' and 'illness' are not sharply distinct is that science, if it is to make progress in psychological medicine, must take account of, must find ways either of accommodating or of accommodating to, concepts such as these.

Note that this is not a retreat from science. Others have argued that a mature psychology, whether medical or general, should incorporate accounts *other* than the scientific. One of the founders of scientific psychiatry, Karl Jaspers, made essentially this point in his early paper, "Causal and "meaningful" connexions between life history and psychosis" (1913a). And the need for hermeneutics in psychology, for explanatory schemes couched in terms of the meanings of experience, to stand alongside the causal explanatory schemes of science, has consistently been argued by those in the existential philosophical tradition of continental Europe. Wulff, Andur Pedersen and Rosenberg (1986) have made a recent contribution to this literature. Furthermore, one specific, if limited, contribution of the present analysis is to provide a single conceptual framework for medicine within which hermeneutic and causal explanations, if not reducible one to the other, or in some other way fully reconcilable, are at least complementary. But what is suggested here – as a speculation, but as a speculation arising directly from the present ethics-based view of medicine – is that the concept of 'action', and with it 'intention', basic as these concepts are to the concept of 'illness', could well be important in the future development of psychology, not adjacently to the science in the subject, as it were, but as part of it.

Note also that this is not a dilution of science. Again, others have argued that psychological science is a diluted science. The so-called post-empiricist philosophers of science have taken much this line, suggesting that psychological science, because relatively value-laden, is more remote from the paradigm science, physics, than is, say, biology. Hesse (1980), for example, having identified a "pragmatic" criterion as the hallmark of physical science, goes on to suggest that by contrast, the sciences of man may be constrained to some extent by quite different values and goals. And in so far as post-empiricism shows science, and medical science in particular, to be embedded in a matrix of value-laden choices, decisions and objectives, social and individual, it of course coincides with the present ethics-based view. Ethical theory, drawing directly on the logic of value-terms, is better placed to put detailed flesh on the bones of this idea. (The analysis of 'disease' set out in chapter 4 provides an example of this.) But as to the idea itself, the two philosophies, coming as it were from opposite directions, nicely cross-reference.

However, on the particular point at issue here, on the closeness of the relationship between psychological science and physics, where post-empiricism tends to push the two disciplines apart, ethical theory, paradoxically, tends to draw them closer together. This is because, if – for the admittedly speculative reason given – psychological science, in order to progress, must find ways either of accommodating or of accommodating to such concepts as 'action' and 'intention', so also, it would seem – though still for speculative reasons – must physics. During most of this century it has been clear that at the level of their conceptual development, there are parallels of a general kind between psychology and physics. At the heart of quantum mechanics in particular, although one of the most successful physical theories ever, there are deep dilemmas, as there are in psychology, about the relationship between subject and object, observer and observed. Einstein regarded these dilemmas as an indication of the incompleteness of quantum mechanics. Bohr, on the other hand, whose views have become more widely accepted, regarded them as requiring radical changes in our understanding of the nature of reality. And with recent experimental results, notably those of Aspect (1986), strongly supporting Bohr's view, the concepts at issue in the Bohr–Einstein debate have come to look uncannily like those at issue in the mental-illness debate (as interpreted on our present ethics-based view). Bell, for example, whose mathematical analysis of the Bohr–Einstein debate provided the theoretical foundation for Aspect's experiments, speaks of the problem of the relationship between a measuring instrument and the measurer in images clearly reminiscent of those used here in chapter 7 in talking of the relationship between 'function' and 'action' (Bell, 1986). And measuring instruments, after all, are a species of functional object. So that it is perhaps no coincidence that the theoretical physicist d'Espagnat, directly echoing our chapter 6 analysis of functional objects in terms of the intentions of their designers, should conclude that Bohr's interpretation of quantum mechanics "ultimately defines (measuring) instruments in terms of our desires" (1976, p. 95).

The point, of course, is not that these speculations in physics will necessarily prove correct – Bohr's interpretation of quantum mechanics, though standard, and though now supported by hard experimental results, is anyway not universally accepted. The point is rather that the concepts at issue in physical science, and around which these speculations have been generated, are the same as, or at any rate overlap extensively with, those which are shown by an ethics-based view of medicine to be at issue in psychological science. The two sciences, physical and psychological, are in this way parallel. Hence it is that, on this point, psychological science, by being brought that much closer to physics, is not diluted by an ethics-based view, but, on the contrary, strengthened. And hence it is that this second reason for believing that an ethics-based view of medicine has a positive role to play in promoting scientific advance, though certainly more speculative than the first, is also the more intriguing.

But now it may be said, if this second reason thus involves neither a retreat from nor a dilution of science in medicine, surely it must imply that everything (in medicine) comes back to science after all. And certainly there is a tension here. For the main theme of this book has been that there is more to medicine than science, importantly, nay primarily, *evaluation*. And the evaluative element in medicine has been traced through 'illness' to the intentionality latent in ' "ordinary" doing', itself a species of 'intentional action'. Yet it now appears that these same, or very similar, concepts have emerged at the heart not merely of psychological but also of physical *science*. At the very least then this must seem like having one's cake and eating it. Either the main theme of the book is correct but this point – here and in physics – is wrong; that is, the concepts of 'intention' and 'action' are after all not really there at the heart of either science. Or the point is right – these concepts really are there – but the main theme of the book is wrong; that is, the medical concepts are either not derived from 'intention' and 'action', or, though they are so derived, they (and with them the medical concepts also) are not, as has here centrally been claimed, essentially value-laden.

Now, the first thing to notice about this tension is that it is not confined to the present ethics-based view. It is also there, to the extent that the arguments showing the value-laden nature of 'intention' are sound, in physics – and d'Espagnat's choice of words, writing of "desires" rather than "intentions", makes it explicit. ("Desires" is italicized in the original.) Then again, it is also there in post-empiricist accounts of science. Kuhn, apparently, has been misread as suggesting that in science might is right, that is, as suggesting that not only the direction of scientific research, but also scientific knowledge as such, what actually counts as scientific "truth", is determined not by the way the world is, but by how this or that social power group wishes or thinks it ought to be (Kuhn, 1970). And Hesse, more moderately, has shown how the relativism implicit in post-empiricist accounts of science has led to a kind of post-post-empiricist realist backlash (Hesse, 1980, p. XIV).

But the second thing to notice about this tension is that it, or something very like it, has already been encountered in this book, and (in principle) resolved – namely, in chapter 10, in the account given of the kind of theory of 'delusion' required to accommodate the full range of the clinical phenomenology of that concept. And chapter 10 holds lessons for us here. Thus, in chapter 10 it seemed at first that the conceptual difficulties presented by the clinical phenomenology of delusions might be resolved by a descriptivist manœuvre, by reducing delusional value judgements to delusional factual judgements, thereby allowing the former to be considered "false" in essentially the same sense as the latter. And post-empiricism in the philosophy of science, to the extent of its relativist implications, can now be seen to be a kind of reciprocal of descriptivism in ethics; the post-empiricist's reduction of facts to values being the reciprocal of the descriptivist's reduction of values to facts.

In chapter 10, however, descriptivism failed. In order to encompass the full range of clinical delusions – value judgements and false factual beliefs, but also true factual beliefs and, crucially, the paradoxical delusion of mental illness – in order to encompass all this, a *non*-descriptivist account was found to be required. Which suggests by extension that a corresponding, non-descriptivist account may be required to resolve the tension raised by the "reciprocal" descriptivism implicit in post-empiricism. Here, as in chapter 10, this idea must be understood as no more than a framework for future research. But *as* a framework, the non-descriptivist ideas developed in chapter 10, seem as appropriate here as there; namely, that instead of attempting to reduce either values to facts or facts to values, both should be derived in a two-level logical system from something "over and above", from some common logical parent. Moreover, the best candidate in chapter 10 for this something "over and above" was the structure of our reasons for action. And this, through the logical connection from reasons to intentions pointed out in chapter 10, brings the argument right back to physics! From clinical delusions, then, through post-empiricism to quantum mechanics – a case, if ever there was one, of what Austin (1956–7) called the negative concept "wearing the trousers". For the tension arising from our second reason for believing that an ethics-based view should contribute to scientific progress, and this tension faced squarely in the non-descriptivist way well established in this book, has now led from the clinical phenomenology of the negative concept of 'delusion' not merely to a parallel between psychology and physics (traditionally the softest and the hardest of sciences) but to an actual closing of the gap between them.

Medicine and philosophy

In science, this "wearing of the trousers" effect – the stimulus to our ideas provided by the negative concept – is important mainly in the more philosophical aspects of the subject. Not that its importance should thus be thought to be any the less. Historically, it is here, rather than in experimental science, that much that is most formative in the development of our ideas about the world takes place (Kuhn's famous "paradigm shifts", 1962). Besides which, philosophy and science, though nowadays separately institutionalized, are not sharply distinct activities. But the message of the present section is that when it comes to philosophy proper, at any rate in its relationship with medicine, the negative concept is truly paramount.

This may seem an extravagant claim. After all, the trade between philosophy and medicine in recent years has been mainly the other way, philosophers becoming involved with medical problems rather than vice versa. And to the extent that it is largely with issues of medical ethics that philosophers have been concerned, this has not happened in isolation, but as part of a more general trend or shift in philosophy, a rather remarkable change of direction away from the epistemological questions which have largely occupied philosophers since the seventeenth century, back to a more medieval concern with moral issues. Philosophers have thus seen in medicine, with its burgeoning ethical problems, a fertile field of enquiry. And doctors, too, have by and large welcomed the involvement of philosophers in this area of practice, recognizing the contribution of their peculiarly analytical skills; rigour, consistency, objectivity, and, importantly, the stomach for what Ernst Nagel has called "the obstinate search for clear meaning" (1961). There are, apparently, some two hundred "clinical ethicists" now in post in the United States (IME, 1987).

In other areas of practice, it is true, the relationship between philosophy and medicine has been more tentative. But granted the science-based illusion, this is consistent. For in these other areas, even in such obvious target areas as the classification of psychiatric disorders, it has been assumed that philosophy (in so far as it is distinct from science) had little to offer. There have been notable exceptions. Stengel, for example, emphasized the importance of the philosopher Hempel's contribution to his thinking in the preparation of the report upon which the innovative ICD-8 classification was based (Stengel, 1959; cf. chapter 9 above. Interestingly, two years before the publication of Stengel's report, Hempel gave a paper on operational definitions – published in 1961 – before a combined medical and philosophical meeting chaired by Stengel.) But even so there has been no long-term follow-up involvement of philosophers in this area. Philosophers are not mentioned in the introductions to either ICD-9 or DSM–III. Either philosophers did not contribute to the preparation of these classifications, or their contributions were not thought to be of sufficient weight to merit acknowledgement. Certainly, philosophers have not been involved in the development of ICD-10 (Sartorius, 1988). All this is of course not to deny the number of individual collaborations there have been between philosophers and doctors on questions of theory, not least in the debate about 'mental illness'. But as far as clinical practice is concerned, it is mainly in the area of ethics that philosophy has contributed to medicine, with little or no reciprocal contribution from medicine to philosophy in return.

In the first two parts of this book these trends and tendencies were to some extent reproduced. The argument began with the theoretical issues surrounding the concept of 'mental illness', the "mental-illness debate". But right from the start it was recognized that these issues had been raised by difficulties in the *practice* of medicine, and by non-empirical, and indeed mainly *ethical* difficulties at that. Similarly, the method adopted in chapter 1 was that of logical analysis, analysis of the meanings of the terms by which medicine is defined – 'illness' and 'disease' especially – by close attention to their actual use. This approach, although recognized to be lacking somewhat in glamour, was considered to be a necessary preliminary to any attempt to draw directly on metaphysics, even in such (obviously) relevant areas as the mind–body problem. But by the end of chapter 2 the conclusion had already been reached that, within the general method of logical analysis, the medical terms might most profitably be analysed specifically as *value* terms. Chapter 3 then took the form, openly and deliberately, of an exercise in applied ethical theory, a number of arguments from the "is–ought" debate in ethics being applied more or less unchanged to the debate in medicine about the concept of 'mental illness'. And it was from the results of this exercise – crucially, the result that not only 'illness' but also 'disease' and even 'dysfunction' were indeed best understood, in their central uses in medicine, *as* value terms – it was from this that the argument led on in chapter 4 to an analysis of 'disease' and in chapter 5 to a first approximation to an analysis of 'illness'.

In the third part of the book, however, the picture began to change. The connecting theme was still ethical theory. But it had now become clear that any further analysis of the concept of 'illness' – which had by this point emerged as the root notion in the logical structure of medicine – required that it be considered not merely as a value term, but as a term expressing a particular *kind* of value (namely, negative medical value). And with this change of emphasis the argument moved rapidly into areas of philosophy not standardly part of ethics; the analysis of 'function' in chapter 6, the "philosophy of action" in chapter 7 and so on. Moreover, in these new areas, it was apparent that although there were bodies of philosophical literature relevant to the needs of medical theory, there was nothing in the way of, as it was put, "ready-made" philosophical theory upon which to draw. In chapter 3, it had been possible to draw more or less directly on the "is–ought" debate. But in these later chapters there were no philosophical theories of 'function' or 'action' to be had "off the peg" suited to the issues in medical theory raised by 'dysfunction' and by 'action failure'. On the contrary, in exploring the issues raised by 'dysfunction' and by 'action failure', the argument ran more or less directly into difficulties of a general philosophical nature raised by 'function' and by 'action'.

There was of course nothing in this prejudicial to the argument as such. From the point of view of medical theory it showed simply that difficulties which at first sight appeared parochial, difficulties limited to the logic of medicine, resolved on analysis into difficulties of far wider philosophical significance. And looked at now the other way, therefore, from the point of view of philosophical theory, this showed that the original medical difficulties were of interest not just in their own right, but as particular instances of more general philosophical problems. Particular, and, indeed, illuminating instances. For the analyses of 'dysfunction' and 'action failure' pursued in chapters 6 and 7 from the point of view of medical theory, illuminated, in a small way, 'function' and 'action'; i.e., by showing the evaluative logical element in the meanings of these latter concepts carried by 'intention'. To this small extent, then, even in chapters 6 and 7 the negative concepts were already "wearing the trousers". And this became increasingly the case in subsequent chapters. In chapter 8, for example, the analysis of alcoholism in terms of our by then well developed reverse-view of the logical structure of medicine suggested a novel approach to the philosophical problem of the difference between an irresistible impulse and an impulse which is not resisted (itself part of the "free-will" problem). And in chapter 10, the analysis of 'delusion', again in reverse-view terms, not only showed the need for an extension of non-descriptivist ethical theory, but also suggested how such an extension might be developed. This in turn led, in the preceding subsection of the present chapter, to a corresponding argument in respect of the implications of post-empiricism in the philosophy of science. Then again, the importance of the phenomenology of delusions, and indeed of the medical concepts generally, in relation to our understanding of the concept of "person" was mentioned in chapter 10, in the context of primary health care. And to all these observations it should now be added that the phenomenology of delusions, in particular the parallel status of value judgements and factual judgements *as* delusions, clearly has epistemological implications also; i.e., for our understanding of the "justification" which (classically) converts mere true belief into knowledge. The deluded patient, it seems, fails in what Robert Nozick calls "tracking the truth" (1981); but the sense in which he fails remains to be explored philosophically.

To some extent it was to be expected that the argument would develop this way. It is in the nature of logical analysis that, past a certain point, it tends to break through into metaphysics. This is because problems of meaning, in however restricted an area of ordinary usage, often stem from, and thus are symptomatic of, deeper metaphysical difficulties. And as far as medicine is concerned, the importance of abnormal psychology as a resource for philosophical analysis was anticipated by Austin himself in his "wearing the trousers" article (1956–7). But what is different here is that any breaking through into metaphysics has been correlated, as the argument of the book has developed, not with an increase in the intensity or thoroughness of the philosophy, but rather with a progressive closeness of approach to first-hand clinical experience. This correlation runs through the book as a whole: in parallel with the shift from logical analysis to metaphysics there is a shift from general to increasingly specific references to clinical material. And the correlation comes to a head in chapter 10, in which the momentum with which the argument is driven towards an extension to non-descriptivist ethical theory (and hence in the present chapter towards a corresponding extension to post-empiricism in the philosophy of science) comes directly from the clinical phenomenology of the concept of 'delusion' as illustrated by actual case histories.

It is no exaggeration to say that this correlation is the key to the future of the relationship between philosophy and medicine. It shows, first, as we have just seen, that as a philosophical resource, medicine, and in particular psychological medicine, is a hot spot not just of ethical but also of a whole range of other kinds of philosophical problems. In the future, therefore, medicine should be of interest to philosophers not just for its ethical issues, still less for these issues as problems merely in practical ethics, but for the problems in general philosophy into which these issues, through logical analysis of the medical concepts, resolve. What the correlation also shows, however, is that in order to see these problems for what they are, in order to break through from logical analysis to metaphysics, philosophers must somehow get closer to the primary data, to first-hand clinical experience. This, too, is illustrated by chapter 10. In considering 'delusion', it seems likely that philosophers – Flew, Glover and so on – had failed to take account of either true factual beliefs or of value judgements in the clinical phenomenology of the concept, essentially because they had been obliged to rely on received medical theory (that is, on the standard medical definition of 'delusion' as a false factual belief), rather than on first-hand observations of deluded patients. It is not easy for philosophers to get closer to first-hand clinical experience. Merely "sitting in", even where ethically permissible, is likely to leave the philosopher in effect still seeing the data second-hand, through the philosophically unsophisticated eyes of their medical colleagues. But given the resource which is there, then the correlation between metaphysics and clinical practice – getting closer to the one bringing one closer to the other – provides a strong incentive for philosophers to find ways of getting closer. And if they do get closer, the correlation itself shows that their ambitions in medicine – and indeed the expectations which doctors have of them – can afford to be enlarged well beyond their present preoccupation with medical ethics.

Yet there is more to it than this. For the correlation also shows that as philosophers get closer to first-hand clinical experience, they will find medicine, as a resource, to be no mere passive repository of metaphysical data, but an active catalyst to philosophical theory. In chapter 10, it was the data themselves, the data of delusional phenomenology, at one and the same time clinical and metaphysical data, which were the main constraint on theory. And constraint, notice, not restraint. For, rather as in science, the data in chapter 10 were not inhibitory but facilitatory; they did not hold back the development of theory but channelled and focussed it forwards. The analogy, indeed, is apt. There is, perhaps, more scope with philosophical than scientific enquiries for the data to be adapted to theory rather than theory to the data. This is what happens, after all, when in seeking to resolve confusions and muddles in ordinary usage, logical analysis passes from a descriptive to what Strawson (writing of metaphysics) calls a "revisionary" phase (Strawson, 1959) – the revisions suggested by logical analysis being revisions to ordinary usage itself. But the danger, which is illustrated in chapter 10, is that of premature set, of prematurely dismissing the data of ordinary usage as confusion or muddle merely because it conflicts with established theory.

The dismissal of the term 'psychosis' by some doctors interested in classification, despite its continued active use, is, if the argument of chapter 10 is correct, one example of this. Any tendency to dismiss delusional true factual beliefs and even the more common delusional value judgements as unimportant oddities, or simply as diagnostic errors, would be another and more serious example. For such a tendency would amount to nothing more than an out-and-out attempt to adapt the clinical data – the actual phenomenology of clinical delusions – to the established theory implicit in the standard medical definition of 'delusion'. There might, indeed, have been an argument for changing the *term* used in chapter 10 for clinical delusions, perhaps to 'pathological beliefs' or possibly 'psychotic beliefs' (not all pathological beliefs being psychotic beliefs). This would have avoided the necessity for the use of such convoluted phrases as "delusional delusions" to emphasize the point that not all delusions medically speaking – that is, as symptoms of mental illness – are delusions non-medically speaking – that is, false factual beliefs. And such a change in terminology might indeed one day be appropriate in ordinary clinical usage if the analysis suggested in chapter 10 turns out to be correct. But merely to have dismissed the data would have left wholly untouched the key philosophical question of just why it is that the (current) medical use of 'delusion' denotes not only false factual beliefs but also true factual beliefs and value judgements. Call them what you will, the use of a common medical name for such disparate logical species points to an important family connection among them as species of pathology. And it was in tracing this connection, accepting the data in their own right rather than trying to adapt them to the standard definition, that the argument of chapter 10 broke through to the metaphysical implications of the clinical concept of 'delusion'.

But there is still more. For this constraint, as a catalyst to philosophical theory, is but a first outcome criterion constraint – that is, a constraint on theory (though now not just on medical philosophical theory, as in chapter 1, but on general philosophical theory as well), arising from the requirement that it should clarify ordinary usage. But the correlation between clinical practice and metaphysics shows that general philosophical theory, in so far as it is derived from clinical practice, is also, like medical philosophical theory, subject to a second outcome criterion constraint – namely, to the constraint that it be practically useful. As a constraint on medical philosophical theory, this second outcome criterion constraint came from the fact that the conceptual issues with which the logical analysis of medical terms is concerned were raised originally by difficulties in everyday clinical practice. And the correlation between clinical practice and metaphysics simply takes this a step further. It shows that where problems in the logic of medicine resolve into problems of a general philosophical nature, then clinical utility becomes a test not merely of medical but also of general philosophical theory. Let it be said again, as was said earlier in this chapter of medical philosophy, this is nothing to do with cost–benefit analysis. It is simply that where clinical difficulties resolve by way of logical analysis into general philosophical difficulties, the extent to which philosophical theory helps to clarify the original clinical difficulties is necessarily a test of success. The point is that for philosophy in its relationship with medicine, success – or at any rate progress – is mandatory. And if this were not a sufficient spur to philosophical theory, notice that the correlation between clinical practice and metaphysics leaves the philosopher, in any effective relationship with medicine, face to face with the patient. This is distinctly uncomfortable. It leaves no room for the (surely defensive) conceit that in philosophy elegance and ingenuity are sufficient. These are important, possibly even necessary, virtues. But here they are not sufficient. Here the abstract objects of metaphysical contemplation become, in the data of first-hand clinical experience, the concrete troubles of an individual patient. To the theoretical requirement for progress, therefore, which is the essence of this second outcome criterion constraint, is added the urgency of practical necessity.

In no less than four respects, then, medicine wears the trousers in its relationship with philosophy: in two first outcome criterion respects, since ordinary medical usage (especially in psychological medicine) is both a resource of metaphysical data and a catalyst to philosophical theory, and in two second outcome criterion respects, since clinical utility supplies both a test of theory and, in the person of the patient, the motivation of necessity.

Yet all that having been said, it must now be acknowledged that this has been a somewhat lop-sided presentation of the case. Some balancing up, some recognition of the importance of philosophy to medicine, rather than just of medicine to philosophy, is clearly needed. "Clearly", because the correlation itself, between clinical practice and metaphysics, has two sides to it. One side, the side emphasized here, shows that philosophers need medicine. But the other side, correspondingly, shows that doctors need philosophy. In one sense this is already evident enough. The non-empirical problems of medical practice, with which this book generally has been concerned, although grist for the philosophical mill, remain, none the less, essentially problems of medical practice. But what is shown by the correlation, in relation to problems of this kind, is that if philosophy is ever to make any useful contribution to medical practice, then doctors – not all doctors, of course, but doctors as a profession – must get rather closer to philosophy than they are at present. In chapter 10, in the case of delusions, it was precisely *because* medical eyes are by and large philosophically unsophisticated that philosophers had not been able to see through them to the philosophically relevant clinical data.

What is needed, then, not just in the case of delusions, but for all the further clinical and philosophical results outlined in this chapter and chapter 11, is that, in addition to philosophers moving closer to medicine, doctors move closer to philosophy. What is needed is the development of a hybrid, similar to that existing between medicine and science, a hybrid of equal partners. Not that it will be any easier for doctors to get closer to philosophy than it is for philosophers to get closer to medicine. The necessary philosophical skills, the skills of logical analysis, take time and practice to acquire – like learning mathematics, or perhaps a martial art, rather than, say, history. But the recognition of mutual need is a first step towards the emergence of the required hybrid, a hybrid which, if the arguments developed here are correct, will be more ambitious than either of its thoroughbred parents in the scope of its philosophical enquiries in medicine, more impatient for progress and more optimistic of success.

Appendix

Comparison of conventional and reverse-view interpretations of the properties of the medical concepts in ordinary usage

In this appendix the analysis of the medical concepts developed in the book is compared in tabular form with the conventional view.
This brings out the way in which the present analysis provides a more complete picture of these concepts.

PROPERTIES OF MEDICAL CONCEPTS	INTERPRETATIONS	
	CONVENTIONAL VIEW	REVERSE VIEW
1. DISTINCTIONS BETWEEN CONCEPTS		
1.1 Illness is sometimes synonymous with disease; sometimes distinct (ch. 2)	Generally not addressed (but see 2,3,5, below) (ch. 2)	Reflects use of disease as sub-category of illness (ch. 4)
1.2 Illness is closely linked with dysfunction but never synonymous (because *people* etc. fall ill; but their *bodies/parts* of their bodies fail to function properly: ch. 2, ch. 6)	Not addressed (ch. 2)	Illness is derived from action, dysfunction from function; action is attributed to people etc., function to bodies/parts of bodies (chs. 6 and 7 generally)
2. ILLNESS		
2.1 Illness expresses a negative value judgement distinct from, e.g. moral and aesthetic negative value judgements (ch. 5)	Scope of illness restricted by that of disease (of which it is a subcategory) but see 3.1 below (ch. 2)	Specifically medical value derived via illness from the logical origins of the medical concepts in the experience of action failure (ch. 7)

Appendix (*cont.*)

PROPERTIES OF MEDICAL CONCEPTS	INTERPRETATIONS	
	CONVENTIONAL VIEW	REVERSE VIEW
2.2 Illness is an excuse (morally and in law) (ch. 10)	Illness, as a subcategory of disease = dysfunction, implies incapacity – but see 4.1/2 below (ch. 10)	Status of illness as an excuse derived (primarily) from action failure (ch. 10)
2.3 Compared with disease (and dysfunction) illness is		
(a) more value-laden	(a)	(a) Disease concepts are derived from the
(b) vague (carrying less definite and explicit factual meanings)	(b)	(b) (logically) primitive sense of 'disease' as "a condition
(c) more culturally variable	Illness is an *evaluative* subcategory of disease, i.e. a "serious" disease (ch. 2)	widely
(c)	(c) regarded as an illness" (the subcategory Id, ch. 4)
(d) used more in lay than technical contexts (e.g. more by patients than by doctors)	(d)	(d) Reflects different uses of value judgements and statements of fact generally (ch. 4)

(e) used more of people than of animals; hardly ever of plants; only metaphorically of machines

RELATIONSHIP ILLNESS/DISEASE

3.1 In the relationship between illness and disease, it is possible for patients

(a) to have a disease without being ill (e.g. early asymptomatic cancer) (ch. 2)

(b) to be ill without the particular disease from which they are suffering having been identified (e.g. before seeing a doctor or with a 'new' disease) (ch. 2)

(c) to be ill without having a disease (e.g. with a hangover) (ch. 2)

(e) Not compatible (ch. 2)

(a) Illness is a subcategory of disease (ch. 4)

(b) ⎤ Not compatible with subcategory theory (ch. 4)

(c) ⎦

(e) Reflects different logical "distances" from action failure (ch. 7)

(a) Disease concepts (once defined) capable of being used independently (ch. 4)

(b) ⎤ Disease is (or is derived from) subcategory (Id) of illness (I), where Id = conditions widely regarded as illnesses (ch. 4)

(c) ⎦

Appendix (*cont.*)

PROPERTIES OF MEDICAL CONCEPTS	INTERPRETATIONS	
	CONVENTIONAL VIEW	REVERSE VIEW
4. **RELATIONSHIP ILLNESS/DYSFUNCTION**		
4.1 Disease forms a bridge of meaning between illness and dysfunction, being sometimes synonymous with one, sometimes with the other, sometimes with neither (ch. 2)	Not addressed (ch. 2)	Bridge of meaning formed by series of linked concepts, I (illness) ↔ Id (sub-category of illness = those conditions widely regarded as illnesses = logically primitive senses of disease) ↔ other disease categories defined by relationship *to* Id; includes causal conditions, some of which are dysfunctional conditions (ch. 4)
4.2 In respect of certain conditions (e.g. sudden loss of movement of an arm) illness and dysfunction are equivocal, the condition being capable of being construed either way (ch. 4)	Not addressed (ch. 4)	Not fully explained but corresponds with (and is capable of being explained further in terms of) the equivocation between action and function (ch. 8)

5.	**DISEASE**		
5.1	Diseases are defined variously but especially in terms of (a) symptoms, (b) statistical associations of symptoms, signs etc. (c) causes, especially disturbances of function. Historically, there has been a shift from (a) through (b) to (c) (ch. 2)	All reflect development of scientific medicine leading to a refinement of the *concept* of disease (ch. 2; ch. 9)	Disease theory of 4.1 allows in principle for an indefinitely large variety of disease categories; within this, the categories actually employed depend on empirical (not logical) considerations, viz. which varieties are most useful for given purposes, and the extent of empirical knowledge (especially of causes) available. Historical and diagnostic shifts between disease categories reflect these empirical considerations rather than conceptual refinement (ch. 4)
6.	**DYSFUNCTION**		
6.1	Some, but not all, dysfunctional bodily/ mental conditions are diseases: e.g. disabilities, wounds, being unfit, death. Similarly, dysfunction relates only to things that can ordinarily be done (not e.g. to seeing in ultraviolet) (ch. 2; ch. 6)	Not addressed. Incompatible with "disease = dysfunction" theories (ch. 2)	Not fully explained. However, (a) wounds reflect distinction between illness and things done/happening *to* people etc.; (b) disabilities reflect absence of expectation of change (necessary to experience of failure of "ordinary" doing); death is the extreme case of this (c) being unfit/

Appendix (cont.)

| PROPERTIES OF MEDICAL | INTERPRETATIONS | |
CONCEPTS	CONVENTIONAL VIEW	REVERSE VIEW
7. MENTAL ILLNESS VERSUS PHYSICAL ILLNESS		
7.1 Mental illness more problematic clinically than physical illness (ch. 1)	Mental illness obscure in meaning compared with physical illness (and/or less sound and/or less authentic) (see ch. 1 generally)	Illness *generally* obscure in meaning; its relatively prolematic use in respect of mental-illness constituents, and relatively *un*problematic in respect of physical, reflects the properties of these constituents (cf., 2.3, (a), (b), (c)
7.2 Mental illness compared with physical illness is more value-laden (also relatively vague and culturally variable) (ch. 1)	Mental illness defective compared with paradigm physical illness (ch.1, generally)	Reflect greater (psychological) variability of criteria by which mental illness constituents (anxiety, sadness etc.) are evaluated compared with physical-illness constituents (movement, sensation) (ch. 5, subsection "Requirement 2")

seeing in ultraviolet reflect norms implicit in "ordinary" doing (ch. 7)

7.3	'Action failure' more prominent in definitions of mental disorders than of physical (e.g. alcoholism, ch. 8)	Not addressed	Attribution of elements of action more problematic for mental than for bodily actions (e.g. attributions of intentions in respect of desires, re alcoholism, ch. 8, subsection "Requirement 2")
7.4	Illness more prominent in psychological medicine than in physical; disease less prominent (ch. 1)	Reflects primitive stage of development of psychological medicine (ch. 5)	Prominence of illness reflects clinical importance of problems raised by mental illness (see 7.1) (ch. 4) Disease less prominent due to (a) less well-developed (because more difficult) scientific base, (b) more variable evaluative criteria for mental-illness constituents than for bodily, thus leading to relatively fewer mental conditions in disease subcategory Id and the further disease categories derived therefrom (ch. 4, generally)
7.5	Psychological medicine has less well-developed causal theories, especially in terms of dysfunction (ch. 1)	Psychological medicine primitive scientifically; has to catch up physical medicine (ch. 2)	Psychological medicine harder to develop scientifically, for empirical and for conceptual reasons; has to develop independently (ch. 9,

Appendix (*cont.*)

PROPERTIES OF MEDICAL CONCEPTS	INTERPRETATIONS	
	CONVENTIONAL VIEW	REVERSE VIEW
		re classification; ch. 12, subsection "medicine and science")
7.6 Among mental illnesses, psychotic mental illnesses, especially constituted by delusions, are paradigmatic (reliably identifiable; less variable cross-culturally; construed as illness since classical times) (ch. 10)	No satisfactory "dysfunction" definable; hence distinction psychotic/non-psychotic denied (ch. 10)	Psychosis analysed as action failure of a kind qualitatively more profound than any other (a failure of the definition of what is done as distinct from the instrumental failures involved in other species of illness, mental and physical) (ch. 10)
7.7 Delusions, the paradigm psychotic mental-illness symptoms, occur commonly as false factual beliefs, but also as value judgements and even as true factual beliefs (ch. 10)	Conventional definition as "false beliefs . . . etc." capable of analysis as cognitive "dysfunction"; but covers only part of the clinical phenomenology. No explanation why paradigmatic (ch. 10)	Interpretation of psychosis in 7.6 explains (a) why delusion is paradigm psychotic symptom, (b) the full range of its clinical phenomenology. More research is required here, but now in a new direction; viz. concerned with *reasons for action* rather than with *cognitive reasoning* (ch. 10)

7.8	If mental illness is an excuse, psychotic mental illness is paradigmatically so (ch. 10)	Not addressed (distinction being denied); or interpreted via non-specific seriousness (leaving relevant sense of "serious" undefined); or via disturbance of function (inconsistent with the data) (ch. 10)	Fully consistent with, and partly explained by, reverse-view interpretations of psychosis (7.6) and delusion (7.7) (ch. 10)
7.9	Although varying degrees of paternalism appropriate in medical care, it is only for mental illness, especially psychotic, that compulsory treatment of an adult patient of normal intelligence and in their own interests, is ever justified (ch. 10)	Incompatiable with idea that physical illness is paradigmatic (ch. 10)	

Bibliography

Ackrill, J. L. 1973. *Aristotle's ethics*. Faber and Faber.

American Psychiatric Association. 1980. *Diagnostic and statistical manual of mental disorders* (third edition). Washington: American Psychiatric Association.

Anscombe, G. E. M. 1956–7. Intention. *Proceedings of the Aristotelian Society* 57: 321–32. Reprinted in White, A. R. ed. 1968. *The philosophy of action*. Oxford University Press.

Aspect, A. 1986. Ch. 2 in Davies, P. C. W. and Brown, J. R., eds. *The ghost in the atom*. Cambridge University Press.

Austin, J. L. 1956–7. A plea for excuses. *Proceedings of the Aristotelian Society* 57: 1–30. Reprinted in White, A. R., ed. 1968. *The philosophy of action*. Oxford University Press.

Ayer, A. J. 1936. *Language, truth and logic*. Victor Gollancz, London.
    1976. *The Central Questions of Philosophy*. Penguin Books Limited.

Barondess, J. A. 1979. Disease and illness – a crucial distinction. *The American Journal of Medicine* 66: 375–6.

Bebbington, P. E. 1977. Psychiatry: science, meaning and purpose. *Brit. J. Psychiat.* 130: 222–8.

Bell, J. 1986. Ch. 3 in Davies, P. C. W. and Brown, J. R., eds. *The ghost in the atom*. Cambridge University Press.

Belk, W. P. and Sunderman, F. W. 1947. A survey of the accuracy of chemical analyses in clinical laboratories. *Am. J. Clin. Path.* 19: 853–61.

Bloch, S. 1981. The political misuse of psychiatry in the Soviet Union. Ch. 18 in Bloch, S. and Chodoff, P., eds. *Psychiatric ethics*. Oxford University Press.

Boorse, C. 1975. On the distinction between disease and illness. *Philosophy and Public Affairs* 5: 49–68.
    1976. What a theory of mental health should be. *J. Theory Social Behaviour* 6: 61–84.

Butler, Rt. Hon., the Lord. 1975. Chairman, Report of the Committee on Mentally Abnormal Offenders, Cmnd., 6244. London: Her Majesty's Stationery Office.

Butterworth, J. S. and Reppert, E. H. 1960. Auscultatory acumen in the general medical population. *Journal of the American Medical Association* 174: 32–4.

Campbell, E. J., Scadding, J. G. and Roberts, R. S. 1979. The concept of disease. *Brit. Med. J.* 2: 757–62.

Clare, A. 1979. The disease concept in psychiatry. In Hill, P., Murray, R., Thorley, A. eds. *Essentials of postgraduate psychiatry.* New York: Academic Press, Grune and Stratton.

Cooper, J. E., Kendell, R. E., Gurland, B. J., Sharpe, L., Copeland, J. R. M. and Simon, R. 1972. *Psychiatric diagnosis in New York and London.* Maudsley Monograph No. 20. London: Oxford University Press.

Culver, C. M. and Gert, B. 1982. *Philosophy in medicine: conceptual and ethical issues in medicine and psychiatry.* Oxford University Press.

DSM–III: see American Psychiatric Association, 1980.

Duff, A. 1977. Psychopathy and moral understanding. *Am. Phil. Quart.* 14 (3): 189–200.

Edwards, R. B. 1981. Mental health as rational autonomy. *The Journal of Medicine and Philosophy* 6: 309–22.

Engelhardt, H. T., Jr.: 1975. The concepts of health and disease. In Engelhardt, H. T., Jr. and Spicker, S. F. eds. *Evaluation and explanation in the biological sciences.* Dordrecht, Holland: D. Reidel.

1986. Clinical complaints and the ens morbi. *The Journal of Medicine and Philosophy* 11: 207–14.

Enoch, M. D., Trethowan, W. H. and Barker, J. C. 1967. *Some uncommon psychiatric syndromes.* Bristol: John Wright and Sons.

d'Espagnat, B. 1976. *Conceptual foundations of quantum mechanics* (second edition). W. A. Benjamin, Inc.

Etter, L. E., Dunn, J. P., Kammer, A. G., Osmond, L. H. and Reese, L. C. 1960. Gastroduodenal X-ray diagnosis: a comparison of radiographic techniques and interpretations. *Radiol.* 74: 766–70.

Eysenck, H. J. 1952. The effects of psychotherapy: an evaluation. *J. Consult. Psychol.* 16 (5): 319–24. Reprinted as Ch. 21 in Eysenck, H. J. and Wilson, G. D. eds. 1973. *The experimental study of Freudian theories.* London: Methuen.

1960. Classification and the problem of diagnosis. Ch. 1 in Eysenck, H. J. ed. *Handbook of abnormal psychology.* London: Pitman Medical Publishing Company Ltd.

Fairburn, C. 1988. Personal communication.

Farrell, B. A. 1979. Mental illness: a conceptual analysis. *Psychological Medicine* 9: 21–35.

1981. *The standing of psychoanalysis.* Oxford University Press.

Fingarette, H. 1972. Insanity and responsibility. *Inquiry* 15: 6–29.

Flew, A. 1973. *Crime or disease?* New York: Barnes and Noble.

Foot, P. 1958–9. Moral Beliefs. *Proceedings of the Aristotelian Society* 59: 83–104. Reprinted in Foot, P. ed. 1967. *Theories of ethics.* Oxford University Press.

Foucault, M. 1973. *Madness and civilization: a history of insanity in the age of reason.* New York: Random House.

Fulford, K. W. M. 1987. Is medicine a branch of ethics? Ch. 8 in Peacocke, A. and Gillett, G., eds. *Persons and personality.* Oxford: Basil Blackwell Ltd.

Gelder, M. G., Gath, D. and Mayou, R. 1983. *Oxford textbook of psychiatry.* Oxford University Press.

Gillon, R. 1985. *Philosophical medical ethics.* Chichester: John Wiley and Sons.

1986. On sickness and on health. *Brit. Med. J.* 292: 318–20.

Glover, J. 1970. *Responsibility.* London: Routledge & Kegan Paul.

Hare, E. H. 1973. A short note on pseudo-hallucinations. *Brit. J. Psychiat.* 122: 469–76.

Hare, R. M. 1952. *The language of morals.* Oxford University Press.

1963a. Descriptivism. *Proceedings of the British Academy* 49: 115–34. Reprinted in Hare, R. M. 1972. *Essays on the moral concepts.* London: The Macmillan Press Ltd.

1963b. *Freedom and reason.* Oxford University Press.

1978. Personal communication.

1981a. *Moral thinking: levels, methods and point.* Oxford: Clarendon Press.

1981b. The philosophical basis of psychiatric practice. Ch. 3 in Bloch, S. and Chodoff, P. eds. *Psychiatric ethics.* Oxford University Press.

Harré, R. and Lamb, R., eds. 1986. *The dictionary of physiological and clinical psychology.* Oxford: Basil Blackwell Ltd.

Hart, H. L. A. 1968. *Punishment and responsibility: essays in the philosophy of law.* Oxford University Press.

Helman, C. G. 1981. Disease versus illness in general practice. *J. Roy. Coll. Gen. Pract.* 230 (3): 548–52.

Hempel, C. G. 1961. Introduction to problems of taxonomy. Pp. 3–22 in Zubin, J. ed. *Field studies in the mental disorders.* New York: Grune and Stratton.

1965. *Aspects of scientific explanation and other essays in the philosophy of science.* New York: The Free Press.

Hemsley, D. R. and Garety, P. A. 1986. The formation and maintenance of delusions: a Bayesian analysis. *Brit. J. Psychiat.* 149: 51–6.

Hesse, M. 1980. *Revolutions and reconstructions in the philosophy of science.* The Harvester Press.

ICD-9: see World Health Organization, 1978.

IME 1987. Clinical ethicists and ethics committees. *Institute of Medical Ethics Bulletin,* Suppl. 5.

Jaspers, K. 1913a. Causal and "meaningful" connexions between life history and psychosis. Ch. 5 in Hirsch, S. R. and Shepherd, M. eds. 1974. *Themes and variations in European psychiatry.* Bristol: John Wright and Sons Ltd.

1913b. *General psychopathology.* Transl. by Hoenig, J. and Hamilton, M. W. 1963. Manchester University Press.

Jellinek, E. M. 1960. *The disease concept of alcoholism.* New Haven, Connecticut: College and University Press.

Jenkins, R. Smeeton, N., Marinker, M. and Shepherd, M. 1985. A study of the classification of mental ill-health in general practice. *Psychol. Med.* 15 (2): 403–9.

Keller, M. 1960. Definition of alcoholism. *Quarterly Journal of Studies on Alcohol.* 21: 125–34.

Kendell, R. E. 1973. The influence of the 1968 glossary on the diagnoses of English psychiatrists. *Brit. J. Psychiat.* 123: 527–30.

1975a. The concept of disease and its implications for psychiatry. *Brit. J. Psychiat.* 127: 305–15.

1975b. *The role of diagnosis in psychiatry.* Blackwell Scientific Publications.

1979. Alcoholism: a medical or a political problem? *Brit. Med. J.* 1: 367–71.

1984. Reflections on psychiatric classification – for the architects of DSM iv and ICD-10. *Integrative Psychiatry* March–April: 43–57.

Kenny, A. J. P. 1969. Mental helath in Plato's republic. *Proceedings of the British Academy* 5: 229–53.

Kuhn, T. S. 1962. *The structure of scientific revolutions* (second edition). *International encyclopedia of unified science.* Vol. 2. No. 2. University of Chicago Press.

1970. Theory-choice. Ch. 15 in Klemke, E. D., Hollinger, R. and Kline, A. D. eds. 1980. *Introductory readings in the philosophy of science.* New York: Prometheus Books.

Laing, R. D. 1967. *The politics of experience.* Harmondsworth: Penguin.

Leff, J. and Isaacs, A. D. 1978. *Psychiatric examination in clinical practice.* Oxford: Blackwell.

Lewis, A. J. 1934. The psychopathology of insight. *Brit. J. Med. Psychol.* 14: 332–48.

1955. Health as a social concept. *Br. J. Sociol.* 4: 109–24.

Lishman, A. W. 1978. *Organic psychiatry.* Oxford: Blackwell Scientific Publications.

1987. Personal Communication.

Lockyer, D. 1981. *Symptoms and illness: the cognitive organization of disorder.* London and New York: Tavistock Publications.

McDowell, J. 1978. Are moral requirements hypothetical imperatives? *Aristotelian Society Proceedings,* Supplementary Volume 52: 13–29.

McGarry, L. and Chodoff, P. 1981. The ethics of involuntary hospitalization. Ch. 11 in Bloch, S. and Chodoff, P., eds. *Psychiatric ethics.* Oxford University Press.

Macklin, R. 1982. Refusal of psychiatric treatment: autonomy, competence, and paternalism. Ch. 6 in Edwards, R. B. ed. *Psychiatry and ethics.* New York: Prometheus Books.

McWhinney, I. R. 1987. Health and disease: problems of definition. *Canadian Medical Assoication Journal* 136: 815.

Maher, B. and Ross, J. S. 1984. Delusions. Ch. 14 in Adams, H. E. and Suther, P. *Comprehensive handbook of psychology.* New York: Plenum Press.

Mayou, R. and Hawton, K. 1986. Psychiatric disorder in the general hospital. *Brit. J. Psychiat.* 149: 172–90.

Melden, A. I. 1959. *Rights and right conduct.* Blackwell.

Mellor, C. S. 1970. First rank symptoms of schizophrenia. *Brit. J. Psychiat.* 117: 15–23.

Menninger, K. 1963. *The vital balance: the life process in mental health and illness.* New York: Viking Press.

Merskey, H. 1986. Variable meanings for the definition of disease. *J. Med. Phil.* 11: 215–32.

Muir Gray, J. A. 1985. The ethics of compulsory removal. Ch. 4 in Lockwood, M., ed. *Moral dilemmas in modern medicine.* Oxford University Press.

Mullen, P. 1979. Phenomenology of disordered mental function. Ch. 2 in Hill, P., Murray, R. and Thorley, A. eds. *Essentials of postgraduate psychiatry.* London: Academic Press. New York: Grune & Stratton.

Nagel, E. 1961. *The structure of science.* Routledge & Kegan Paul.

Nozick, R. 1981. *Philosophical explanations.* Oxford University Press.

Parsons, T. 1951. *The social system.* Glencoe, Illinois: Free Press.

PSE: see Wing *et al.,* 1974.

Quinton, A. 1985. Madness. Ch. 2 in Griffiths, A. P., ed. *Philosophy and practice.* Cambridge University Press.

Rachman, S. J. 1983. Irrational thinking, with special reference to cognitive therapy. *Advances in Behaviour Research and Therapy* 5: 63–88.

Rachman, S. J. and Philips, C. 1978. *Psychology and medicine*. Penguin Books.

Reznek, L. 1987. *The nature of disease*. London and New York: Routledge & Kegan Paul.

Risso, M. and Boker, W. 1968. Delusions of witchcraft: a cross-cultural study. *Brit. J. Psychiat.* 114: 963–72.

Roth, L., Meisel, A. and Lidz, C. W. 1977. Tests of competency to consent to treatment. *Am. J. Psychiat.* 134 (3): 279–84.

Roth, M. 1976. Schizophrenia and the theories of Thomas Szasz. *Brit. J. Psychiat.* 129: 317–26.

Roth, M. and Kroll, J. 1986. *The reality of mental illness*. Cambridge University Press.

Sartorius, N. 1988. Personal communication.

Sedgwick, P. 1973. Illness – mental and otherwise. *The Hastings Studies Center Studies* 1, 3: 19–40 – Institute of Society, Ethics and the Life Sciences, Hastings-on-Hudson, New York.

Shepherd, M. 1961. Morbid jealousy: Some clinical and social aspects of a psychiatric syndrome. *J. Mental Science* 107: 687–704.

Shepherd, M., Cooper, B., Brown, A. C. and Kalton, G. W. 1966. *Psychiatric illness in general practice*. London: Oxford University Press.

Skegg, K. 1978. Personal communication.

Slater, E. 1973. The psychiatrist in search of science. II: Developments in the logic and the sociology of science. *Brit. J. Psychiat.* 122: 625–36.

Stengel, E. 1959. Classification of mental disorders. *Bulletin of the World Health Organisation* 21: 601–63.

Stevenson, C. L. 1937. The emotive meaning of value terms. *Mind* 46: 14–31.

Strawson, P. F. 1959. *Individuals: an essay in descriptive metaphysics*. London: Methuen, University Paperbacks.

Szasz, T. S. 1960. The myth of mental illness. *American Psychologist* 15: 113–18.

1963. *Law, liberty and psychiatry: an inquiry into the social uses of mental health practices*. New York: Macmillan.

Taylor, F. K. 1981. On pseudo-hallucinations. *Psychological Medicine*: 265–72.

1983. A logical analysis of disease concepts. *Comprehensive Psychiatry* 24 (1): 35–48.

Teasedale, J. D., Taylor, R. and Fogarty, S. J. 1980. Effects of induced elation–depression on accessibility of memories of happy and unhappy experiences. *Behaviour Research and Therapy* 18: 339–46.

Thomas, C. S. 1984. Dysmorphophobia: a question of definition. *Brit. J. Psychiat.* 144: 513–16.

Toulmin, S. 1980. Agent and patient in psychiatry. *International Journal of Law and Psychiatry* 3: 267–78.

Urmson, J. O. 1950. On grading, *Mind* 59: 145–69.

Vauhkonen, K. 1968. *On the pathogenesis of morbid jealousy, with special reference to the personality traits of and interaction between jealous patients and their spouses.* Copenhagen: Munksgaard.

Walker, N. 1967. *Crime and insanity in England.* Edinburgh University Press.

1985. Psychiatric explanations as excuses. Ch. 9 in Roth, M. and Bluglass, R. eds. *Psychiatry, human rights and the law.* Cambridge University Press.

Warnock, G. J. 1967. *Contemporary moral philosophy.* London and Basingstoke: The Macmillan Press Ltd.

Warnock, M. 1978. *Ethics since 1900* (third edition). Oxford University Press.

Williams, B. 1985. *Ethics and the limits of philosophy.* Fontana.

Williams, P. and Strauss, R. 1950. Drinking patterns of Italians in New Haven. Utilization of the personal diary as a research tool. *Quarterly Journal of Studies on Alcohol* 11: 51–91, 250–308, 452–83, 586–629.

Winch, P. 1972. Nature and convention. Pp. 50–73 in Winch P. *Ethics and Action.* Routledge.

Wing, J. K. 1978. *Reasoning about madness.* Oxford University Press.

Wing, J. K., Cooper, J. E. and Sartorius, N. 1974. *Measurement and classification of psychiatric symptoms.* Cambridge University Press.

Wittgenstein, L. 1958. *Philosophical investigations* (second edition). Transl. by Anscombe, G. E. M. Oxford: Basil Blackwell Publisher Limited.

Wootton, B. 1959. *Social science and social pathology.* London: George Allen and Unwin.

World Health Organization. 1948. *Manual of the international statistical classification of diseases, injuries and causes of death* (ICD-6). Geneva: WHO.

1967. *Manual of the international statistical classification of diseases, injuries and causes of death* (ICD-8). Geneva: WHO.

1978. *Mental disorders: glossary and guide to their classification in* accordance with the ninth revision of the International classification of diseases. Geneva: WHO.

Wulff, H. R. 1976. Rational diagnosis and treatment. Oxford: Basil Blackwell.

Wulff, H. R., Pedersen, S. A. and Rosenberg, R. 1986. Philosophy of medicine, an introduction. Oxford: Blackwell Scientific Publications.

Index

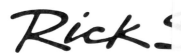
Rick

EASTERN
EUROPE

Rick Steves & Cameron Hewitt

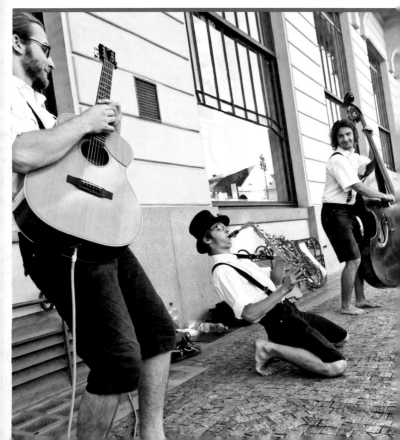

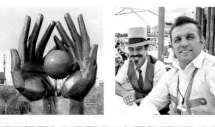
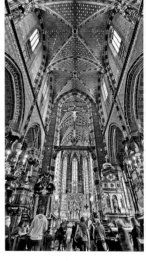
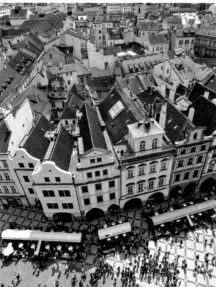
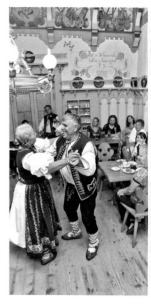
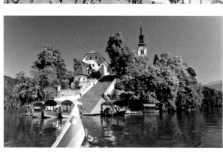
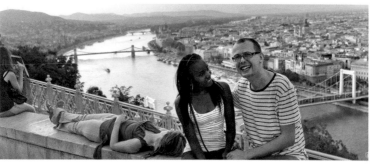